Health Care Cost Containment

Johns Hopkins Studies in Health Care Finance and Administration

Health Care Cost Containment

Karen Davis, PH.D.,
Gerard F. Anderson, PH.D.,
Diane Rowland, SC.D., and
Earl P. Steinberg, M.D., M.P.P.

The Johns Hopkins University Press
Baltimore and London

1990

© 1990 The Johns Hopkins University Press
Printed in the United States of America

The Johns Hopkins University Press
701 West 40th Street
Baltimore, Maryland 21211
The Johns Hopkins Press Ltd., London

The paper used in this publication meets
the minimum requirements of American National
Standard for Information Sciences—
Permanence of Paper for Printed Library
Materials, ANSI Z39.48-1984.

Library of Congress Cataloging-in-Publication Data

Health care cost containment / Karen Davis . . . [et al.].
    p.   cm. — (Johns Hopkins studies in health care finance and
administration : 3)
    Includes bibliographical references.
    ISBN 0-8018-3874-6 (alk. paper). — ISBN 0-8018-3875-4 (pbk.
alk. paper)
    1. Medical care, Cost of—United States—History. 2. Medical
care—United States—Cost control. 3. Medical policy—United
States. I. Davis, Karen, 1942– . II. Series.
    [DNLM: 1. Cost Control—trends—United States. 2. Health
Services—economics—United States. 3. Quality of Health Care—
economics—United States.   W1 J0159H v. 3 / / W 74 H434]
RA410.53.H4143 1989
338.4'33621'0973—dc20
DNLM/DLC   89-45481
for Library of Congress   CIP

Contents

Acknowledgments

The authors wish to thank the Robert Wood Johnson Foundation for funding this work. Drew Altman, Ph.D., who was a vice president at Robert Wood Johnson at the time, originally suggested the need for such a book. The authors express special appreciation to Carl J. Schramm, Ph.D., J.D., for his remarkable vision of the health system and the keen analytic insights he contributed in working sessions throughout the course of the study. They also wish to thank Steven Renn, J.D., for assistance with the review of state rate-setting experience, investigation of the development of preferred provider organizations, and analytic work on the impact of cost containment interventions. The authors thank Joel Cantor, Sc.D., Jennifer Edwards, M.H.S., Jane Erickson, M.H.S., Paula Grant, M.H.S., Sandra Graziano, Ph.D., Robert Herbert, M.S., Denise Hynes, M.P.H., Christina Johns, and Barbara Lyons, M.H.S., for able research assistance, Joanne Allen for editorial assistance, and Yael Fletcher and Marie Davidson for assistance with preparing the manuscript.

The views expressed in this book are those of the authors and do not necessarily reflect those of the Robert Wood Johnson Foundation or the Johns Hopkins University.

Health Care Cost Containment

Chapter 1　**Containing Health Care Costs: Market Competition versus a Coordinated Public Policy**

The U.S. health care system has been characterized by rapidly rising expenditures for several decades. Health expenditures as a percentage of the Gross National Product rose from 4.4 percent in 1950 to 11.2 percent in 1987 (HCFA 1987b). Rapid increases in hospital expenditures—hospitals make up the largest component of the health sector—have been especially troublesome. In 1950 the cost of an average hospital stay was $127; by 1986 this had increased to $3,527 (House Committee on Ways and Means 1988).

Attempts to curb rising costs, to put pressure on the industry to achieve greater productivity or efficiency, and to assure that medical care provided is of genuine value in improving health or patient satisfaction have been sporadic and, with a few notable exceptions, largely unsuccessful. Frustration at the seeming inability of the industry to moderate cost increases has led to a multitude of efforts by government bodies and by private sector organizations to force change. The Medicare program, the largest single purchaser of hospital care, has adopted a new system of paying hospitals which, over time, will place enormous pressure on hospitals to modify their behavior and achieve slower increases in the costs of caring for hospitalized patients (Iglehart 1983b). Simultaneously, private health insurance companies and major corporations have instituted a wide array of features in employee health benefit plans designed to curb rising employer outlays for health services received by employees, dependents, and retirees (Fox, Goldbeck, and Spies 1984). State governments have instituted new ways to pay hospitals under Medicaid programs and have sought to limit their financial liability for health care provided to groups of covered poor (Iglehart 1983a). These efforts, which have surfaced with stunning speed in the early 1980s, are fragmented and lack any cohesive guiding policy.

The long-term implications of the cost containment measures that have been put in place have not been carefully analyzed. Nor has a systematic

1

effort been made to ensure that the measures instituted are consistent with broad social goals, such as promoting and protecting the health of the nation, assuring the provision of quality health care for all, including the poor and the disadvantaged, or seeing that dollars spent on health care result in the maximum health benefit.

Moreover, these efforts come at a time when the capacity of the health sector to provide services has been burgeoning. The supply of physicians is growing rapidly as a result of increases in the number of medical schools since 1960, expansion in medical school class sizes, and an influx of foreign-trained physicians, including U.S. citizens trained in other countries. There has been a major expansion in the number of hospital beds as hospital management anticipated an unending boom in demand and attempted to expand and modernize capital plant and equipment to offer the latest technology to an ever-expanding patient population. The attraction of revenues from public programs and private insurance plans has led to greater investments by for-profit companies in the health sector (Renn et al. 1985). Management innovations have resulted in major chains of hospitals, new cooperative relationships among hospitals, and diversification of the services offered by hospitals in the past (K. Davis 1986).

The speed with which these changes are occurring and the absence of current, comprehensive information have limited public understanding of their implications. For example, very little debate accompanied passage of the changes in Medicare payment policies. Changes are taking place without any guiding public policy other than a general laissez-faire attitude and without any informed public debate about their long-term implications or desirability.

The federal government, which has played a central role in establishing the framework for health policy in the United States in the last two decades, has narrowed its focus. The federal health policy is shaped almost exclusively by federal economic and budgetary policies, which have only one central objective: to limit federal outlays for health services (Blendon 1986a). This policy is mitigated somewhat by a desire by the Congress to protect the poor and elderly directly from the financial brunt of budgetary cutbacks in health services. The major thrust of legislative action, therefore, has been directed at providers, principally hospitals, and has resulted in curbs on payments to providers for services rendered to beneficiaries of Medicare and Medicaid, the two major governmental health financing programs.

This preoccupation with public expenditures for health care of the poor and the elderly can easily lead to a distortion in overall health policy (Blendon and Rogers 1983). It can lead over time to discrimination against patients covered under public programs as their care becomes less "profitable" than care provided to other patients. It can lead to a deterioration in the quality of care for all patients as resources are arbitrarily constrained to meet budget objectives. It can lead to the sacrifice of other public goals, such as ensuring access to health care for the most vulnerable members of society, supporting biomedical research to conquer disease, enhancing the quality of health care, and safeguarding and improving the health of the nation—with little public understanding that this tradeoff is occurring or public agreement that it should occur.

The environment in which cost containment measures are being instituted raises special concerns. Unlike most other industrialized nations, the United States does not have a national health insurance system that provides universal coverage to the entire population and guarantees a minimum level of health care for all (Blendon, Altman, and Kilstein 1983; Davis 1975). Instead the United States has a patchwork system of public and private health insurance coverage that leaves 37 million Americans without any health insurance coverage (Census 1987a). The charitable impulses of providers that created free or discounted care have given way in many instances to an emphasis on businesslike attitudes, attention to the "bottom line," and the need to survive in a cut-throat competitive environment.

Health care for those who cannot pay, therefore, becomes a "hot potato," with transfers from one hospital to another occurring because the patient has no insurance (Schiff et al. 1986). Public institutions have limited budgets and operate under policies that require them to turn away patients from other jurisdictions. No genuine safety net exists in the United States to assure that those in need of health care receive it—through adequate insurance coverage, a network of public hospitals and clinics, or charity care.

Superimposition of a set of financial incentives that encourages institutions to cut costs and protect their financial position in the absence of such a safety net creates the danger that cost containment measures will be felt by those least able to cope with such stringency. Rather than respond to financial incentives by improving productivity and efficiency, eliminating marginally beneficial services, or curbing excess managerial and professional salaries or profits, providers may simply refuse to see charity patients, discriminate against less profitable patients, such as those frail elderly who require extensive nursing assistance or have complicating conditions, and slow down the adoption of costly technology despite its long-term potential contribution to health improvement. Clearly, this response very likely is not what was intended by the designers of innovative approaches to contain costs, but without a balanced guiding health policy that stresses the full panoply of social goals, such a response is not only possible but perhaps probable.

This does not mean that efforts to contain health care costs should be abandoned. It does mean that such efforts need to be carefully scrutinized to determine their effectiveness and any harmful effects. Modification of these approaches may need to be instituted to correct the most serious failings. A public consensus about a blueprint for the health sector consonant with broad social goals becomes especially imperative in this environment (Blendon and Altman 1984).

Why Are Health Care Costs a Concern?

Rising health care costs are universally believed to be a bad thing. This is quite unlike the case in other sectors of the economy, where greater sales are universally believed to be a good thing. If the health sector were not booming, it might be argued, there would be less real growth in the economy, unemployment would be higher, and the standard of living of the population would be lower.

Why is it, then, that rising health care costs have generated such concern? The basic reason is a belief that spending on health care does not generate benefits in terms of improved health or patient satisfaction commensurate with the resources required to provide the care (Fuchs 1974).

Efficiency and Profits

This general belief can be expressed more technically in terms of inefficiency (Feldstein 1988). *Allocative efficiency*, that is, the allocation of a nation's resources in such a way as to generate the "right" (most valued) mix of outputs, is a goal of most economies. There is concern in the United States that too many health services are produced. This concern is based on the allegation that real spending on health care has increased without evidence of commensurate increases in health improvement or patient satisfaction. It is argued that excess surgery takes place and that patients receive laboratory or radiological tests because of physician curiosity or concern with malpractice rather than because they contribute to improved diagnosis or treatment. Indeed, some health care services provided are harmful, not beneficial, and other services provide only minimal benefits. The personnel, capital, and other resources now devoted to producing these services could, it is argued, be better diverted to producing other goods and services. Fewer nurses and more teachers could be trained. Fewer hospitals could be built, and more roads repaired.

Translating the concept of allocative efficiency into monetary terms, if employees used fewer hospital services, employee health insurance premiums would be lower and employers could afford to pay workers higher wages, to pay stockholders higher dividends, or to charge consumers lower prices. In turn these higher wages, dividends, or savings could be used privately to purchase whatever those workers, stockholders, or consumers preferred. If the use of unnecessary health services by the elderly and poor were reduced, federal and state governmental budgets would be reduced, resulting in lower taxes, more funds for other public priorities, or reduced deficits and diversion of capital borrowing from private uses.

A second concern is that the health services provided in the United States are not produced at the lowest cost, that is, that the health care sector does not attain *productive efficiency*. Having costly specialists provide primary care that could be provided more cheaply by primary care physicians and having physicians provide services that could be provided equally well by nurses or nurse practitioners are examples of productive inefficiency. Having an uncomplicated pregnancy handled in a complex, highcost teaching hospital with specialized personnel in attendance may also be viewed as an unnecessarily costly way of providing health care.

A third concern is that the lack of competition in the health care sector leads to excess profits, including higher incomes for physicians and hospital owners than would be earned in a perfectly competitive free market.

Public Acceptability

A desire to reduce the financial burdens of health care expenses underlies public support for cost containment measures (Blendon and Altman 1984). Most Americans are, however, reasonably satisfied with the care they receive and unwilling to make radical changes in the way they receive health care. Public support for cost containment measures tend to be greatest for long-term measures, such as investing in biomedical research or making positive changes in lifestyle. There is support for shorter-term measures that change incentives facing health care providers through competitive or regulatory measures. For the most part there is little support for measures that would increase patient out-of-pocket costs for health care, limit the patient's freedom to choose a physician or hospital, or reduce health care for the poor. Blendon and Altman (1984) argue that this public ambivalence toward health care costs places a premium on a mixed strategy of public and private cost containment.

Pressures for health care cost containment also come from employers concerned with high premiums for employee health benefits. They come from public officials and taxpayers who wish to curb spending under health programs financed by government. Measures acceptable to employers and public officials are also affected by employee attitudes and public opinion.

Public support for cost containment could be expected to be greatest for those measures that have relatively little effect on high-quality essential health care. The difficulty with developing such a cost containment strategy is identifying those health services that yield no or little benefit and developing a system of incentives or regulation that will lead to their elimination, without any reduction in services important to patients and without causing them harm (Blendon and Rogers 1983). In practice, any cost containment measure is likely to affect both highly valued services and less worthwhile services. The challenge is to identify the mix of policies that best preserves health-improving services and eliminates ineffective services.

Equity and Access

Containing health care costs is only one social goal guiding health policy. In his book on the tradeoff between equity and efficiency, Okun notes that "the case for a right to survival is compelling. The assurance of dignity for every member of the society requires a right to a decent existence— to some minimum standard of nutrition, health care, and other essentials of life. Starvation and dignity do not mix well" (Okun 1975). As a society, we are willing to sacrifice some efficiency, if necessary, to assure that all members of society have access to health care and that health services are equitably distributed.

Overview

This book attempts to inform those concerned with the effort to contain health care costs in the United States about the impact and effectiveness of the myriad approaches to health care cost containment launched over the last fifteen years by public bodies and private organizations. It sets forth a long-range policy proposal for change that will ensure the evolution of a health industry that is consistent with broad social goals. The primary emphasis of this book is on examining those approaches that have been tried over the last fifteen years to contain health care costs by changing the financial incentives faced by providers of health care through reform of provider payment methods. Altering financial incentives, it is believed, could induce physicians, hospital managers, and others to choose those services that are most effective and most beneficial.

The rationale for a provider payment reform strategy is the conviction that the best sorting out of high- and low-benefit services will come from professional judgment by those providing the care. This strategy places less reliance on individual patients deciding which services are important than would a strategy based on restructuring the extent to which patients share in the cost of their health care bills. It also does not rely heavily on public officials' judgments about the importance of individual services, as a strategy emphasizing primarily health planning or supply controls would.

Provider payment reform has been tried in a number of guises. Financial incentives through provider payment provisions have been implemented in the Medicare and Medicaid programs, which finance health services for the elderly and poor. Others have been instituted by state governments through statewide rate-setting provisions. Private sector approaches have grown in importance in recent years and include encouragement of employees to enroll in health maintenance organizations (HMOs) or preferred provider organizations (PPOs), which offer price discounts to employers.

Chapter 2 reviews public and private approaches to health care cost containment as public policy slowly evolved from a concern with assuring access to health care and an adequate supply of health professionals and facilities to a concern with excessive health care costs. It details federal legislative attempts to place mandatory limits on increases in hospital revenues in 1977 and the hospital industry's response that private voluntary efforts would be sufficient to bring cost increases in line with social objectives. Legislative consideration of mandatory hospital cost controls in the late 1970s was important analytically and politically in establishing the need for and developing promising approaches to more concerted efforts in the early 1980s.

Chapter 3 turns to federal cost containment efforts in the early 1980s, with a discussion of the provisions of the Tax Equity and Fiscal Responsibility Act of 1982 (TEFRA), which changed hospital payment under Medicare, and the Diagnosis-Related Group Prospective Payment System, enacted in 1983.

Chapter 4 examines state government approaches to cost containment under the Medicaid program, including major shifts in state Medicaid hospital payment practices following enactment of legislation in 1981 freeing states from following Medicare hospital payment policy and encouraging states to manage care of beneficiaries by contracting with a restricted set of Medicaid providers. Lessons from a case study of managed care in the Wisconsin Medicaid program illustrate the managerial and quality concerns raised by rapid implementation of managed care systems.

Chapter 5 highlights the experience of state rate-setting agencies in selected states that evolved their own approaches to reviewing hospital budgets or setting rates for services rendered to hospital patients. Empirical evidence on the effectiveness of state rate-setting programs in slowing the rate of increase in hospital costs is presented.

Chapter 6 details the cost containment measures incorporated in corporate employee health benefits plans. It reviews major changes in employee health benefit plans adopted in the early 1980s, including increased patient cost sharing, measures to reduce utilization of hospital services, incentives for employees to enroll in HMOs and PPOs, and programs to promote the health of employees.

Chapter 7 describes one of the major competitive changes that has occurred in the health care market, the expansion of HMOs. It reviews the evolution of HMOs over the period 1970–85, including federal government efforts to encourage HMO growth, and the changing nature of the HMO industry. It summarizes the evidence on HMO performance, including enrollment trends, cost savings, and quality. Lessons from a case study of HMO development in Baltimore highlight the potential, as well as the difficulties and concerns that growth of HMOs hold for public policy.

Chapter 8 examines historical trends in health care costs, with emphasis on the hospital sector. It traces the trends in real health expenditures and real hospital expenditures over the period 1950–85. It presents data on the varying performance of the health sector during periods of rapid growth in private insurance coverage, the introduction of Medicare and Medicaid, the Economic Stabilization Program followed by the removal of controls, the pursuit of hospital cost containment legislation under the Carter administration and the hospital industry's response of a Voluntary Effort to control costs, emergence of the market as a major determinant of costs, and finally the introduction of hospital prospective payment under Medicare.

Chapter 9 examines the impact of cost containment measures on hospital care of the poor. It presents empirical evidence on trends in utilization of hospital services by the uninsured and by the poor covered by Medicaid with the increase in competitive pressures on hospitals and cutbacks in the Medicaid program.

Chapter 10 considers the potential long-term effects of cost containment on the quality of care and sets forth several actions that will need to be taken to guarantee quality under various cost containment approaches.

Chapter 11 summarizes the major lessons to be derived from the multiple approaches to health care cost containment attempted over the period from 1970–85.

Chapter 12 defines a set of social goals that should guide health policy and presents a long-range policy proposal that would expand access to health care services and coordinate provider payment under public and private auspices. This blueprint provides a starting point for widespread public discussion and debate regarding what we want the U.S. health system to achieve and how best to obtain that goal.

It should be noted, however, that the book does not deal directly with one crucial aspect of provider payment—financial incentives for physicians. In large part, this is a reflection of the absence of major interventions to change physician payment methods in the last two decades. The absence of experience with different physician payment innovations is regrettable. Physician services account for 20 percent of all health outlays, but directly or indirectly physicians control over 70 percent of health expenditures through their decisions on which patients to hospitalize and which drugs to prescribe. The predominant mode of physician payment is on a fee-for-service basis. This system of payment gives physicians a financial incentive to expand the services given to patients. Only for physicians providing care in some types of HMOs, PPOs, and teaching hospital arrangements are these incentives neutralized. A broader inquiry into modifying physician behavior through payment reform is clearly warranted, as several major policy reports have indicated (CBO 1986; Jencks and Dobson 1985; OTA 1986). Such an inquiry, however, is beyond the scope of this book.

Chapter 2   **Early Attempts to Control Health Care Costs, 1950–1980**

In contrast to the health care systems in most other industrialized countries, the U.S. health care system uses multifarious revenue sources to finance health care services. Calls for a universal, national health insurance system, including proposals from Presidents Truman, Nixon, Ford, and Carter, have been rejected in favor of retaining a mixed, pluralistic system of health care financing. Health insurance for those in the workforce and their dependents comes primarily from employers. Since 1965 Medicare and Medicaid have provided coverage for many of those outside the workforce. Medicare covers 32 million elderly and disabled people. Medicaid covers 23 million low-income individuals, primarily one-parent families with children, and the disabled and the elderly (HCFA 1987a). About 37 million Americans have no health insurance coverage from any source (Census 1987b).

The absence of a unified health financing system has contributed to a fragmented approach to containing costs in the health care sector. Responsibility for trying to promote efficiency in the health care sector and to contain costs has been shared by both the private and the public sector.

Provisions to slow increases in health care costs are embodied in provider payment methods incorporated in major public and private insurance plans. Medicare cost containment provisions have applied uniformly to care of the elderly, nationwide. In contrast, Medicaid provisions for paying health care providers and incentives for efficiency have varied considerably from one state to another. Employers have independently designed their health benefit plans for employees in accordance with desired corporate objectives and negotiations with unions. States have enacted legislation to curtail health care costs through such measures as health planning or Certificate of Need (CON) laws and in some instances through the creation of state hospital rate or budget review commissions. Federal legislation to support construction of hospitals, training of health professionals, creation of HMOs, and the planning of health services have also affected costs in the health sector.

The following sections examine the forces shaping the financing of health care and the growing interest in health care costs over five distinct time periods spanning the years 1950–80.

The Growth in Private Health Insurance, 1950–1965

Following the end of World War II major social changes occurred in the United States which in turn affected the health sector. The War Labor Board in 1942 established that employer-provided health insurance coverage to workers did not represent a violation of wage controls. Collective bargaining expanded in the late 1940s and early 1950s, and as a result employee health insurance coverage became a negotiable item (Starr 1982). The period following World War II was characterized by expanding health insurance coverage, particularly for workers and their dependents. The private health insurance industry grew from a $1 billion industry in 1950 to an $8.7 billion industry in 1965.

In the late 1940s the American Medical Association opposed the passage of comprehensive national health insurance as proposed by President Truman. However, it did acquiesce to the provision of health insurance coverage by employers (Starr 1982). AMA opposition to a national health insurance scheme was based on the belief that a universal plan would lead to government intervention in the practice of medicine and cost controls on the health sector.

Employers began to provide health insurance coverage for workers and dependents, with gradual improvements in benefits over time. Coverage of inpatient hospital care was followed by coverage of physicians' fees for surgery and other services performed in the hospital. Insurance coverage for services covered in the physician's office came later and was much less extensive than coverage for hospital care. The early history of insurance coverage emphasized care in an inpatient hospital setting. As this type of insurance coverage became more comprehensive, there was a concomitant growth in hospital expenditures (Law 1974). Physicians were compensated at a higher rate for providing care within the hospital, and specialized procedures were paid at particularly high rates. Incomes of surgeons and other specialty physicians outpaced incomes of pediatricians and family physicians.

Blue Cross initially provided insurance based on a community rate: everyone in a particular geographic area paid the same premium (with perhaps some adjustment for age or family size). Commercial insurance companies, on the other hand, adopted the practice of experience rating. Using this system, an employer plan was charged a premium based on the expected health expenditures of that particular group. With competition from commercial companies, Blue Cross was ultimately forced to move to experience rating to avoid losing healthy, low-cost groups.

The trend toward experience rating and coverage through employment created a tremendous void in coverage for the elderly. Most workers lost their health insurance coverage upon retirement (Merriam 1964). These developments led to the creation of Medicare as a means to provide health insurance coverage to the elderly.

Following World War II the public sector initiated a variety of programs to improve the supply of health care services as well as access to them. Congress enacted the Hill-Burton Act in 1947 to subsidize the construction of hospitals. The GI Bill enabled many veterans to attain a college education and to pursue studies in many fields, including medicine. The National Institutes of Health and health manpower legislation encouraged training of physicians that was geared to specialty care and research.

In 1950 states with federal financial assistance began making payments to hospitals, physicians, and other providers of medical care to those on public welfare assistance. By 1960 about forty states were participating, spending half a billion dollars on medical care for the poor (Davis and Schoen 1978). Financial assistance for health care to the poor was greatly expanded with the passage of the Kerr-Mills Act in 1960. The federal share was increased to an open-ended commitment to pay for an established set of services. And what was most important, financing of health care services was extended to the medically needy elderly. By 1965 all states were providing care to the poor, and in forty-seven states there was optional coverage of the medically needy elderly.

With his election in 1964, President Lyndon Johnson proclaimed the need to create a Great Society and rapidly pushed for enactment of a host of social reforms.

Early Medicare and Medicaid, 1966–1971

The passage of Medicare and Medicaid in 1965 heralded a new era for the federal government's role in health care. After assuming responsibility for financing health care services for 50 million elderly and poor Americans, the federal government moved slowly but inevitably into the role of shaping the health care system to achieve greater efficiency and to ensure attainment of important social goals, such as access to health care for all citizens (Davis and Schoen 1978). Actions by the federal government, particularly those affecting Medicare payment policy, also affected Medicaid and in some instances had important ramifications for the entire health care delivery system.

Medicare

Medicare is a federal program that finances hospital, physician, and other acute-care services for the elderly and, since July 1973, the disabled. Medicare comprises two parts: Part A covers hospital, nursing home, and home health services; Part B covers physician services, outpatient hospital services, and limited ambulatory care services. Coverage under Part A is extended automatically to all persons aged sixty-five and over who receive Social Security payments or railroad retirement cash benefits. Medicare is also available to those individuals who have been permanently and totally disabled for two years or more and to persons with end-stage renal disease. About 95 percent of those covered under Part A of Medicare voluntarily enroll in Part B, which requires payment of a premium. Part A is financed by a payroll tax on employers and employees; Part B is financed by general revenues and premium contributions.

Medicare expenditures have risen rapidly throughout the twenty years of the program (Davis and Rowland 1986). As shown in table 2.1, reimbursement for services increased from $4.5 billion in 1967, the first full year of the program, to nearly $78 billion in 1986. Over this period the number of Medicare enrollees increased from 19.5 million aged to 31.8 million aged and disabled.

The major increase in Medicare enrollment occurred in 1973 after the adoption of the Social Security Act Amendments of 1972, which extended Medicare coverage to the permanently and totally disabled and those with renal disease. In 1987 about 3 million Medicare enrollees were covered because of disability, including 47,000 with end-stage renal disease. That same year 29.5 million of Medicare's 32.4 million beneficiaries were sixty-five and over. Approximately 10 percent of all aged enrollees were eighty-five and over, up from 6 percent when the program was implemented in 1966.

Medicare pays primarily for hospital and physician services. Sixty-nine percent of Medicare expenditures in 1986 were for hospital services, 25 percent were for physician services, and the remainder paid for nursing home care, home health care, miscellaneous services, and administrative expenses.

The growth in Medicare expenditures has been a result of the same factors that affect the total health care system: an aging population, inflation in the economy and in medical care prices, expanding technology, and more services per patient. Medicare payments per aged enrollee have increased faster than health expenditures per capita, primarily because of an increase in hospital admissions of the aged, increased services to hospitalized aged patients, and overall inflation in the cost of hospital care.

Table 2.1. Medicare Enrollees, Reimbursements, and Reimbursements per Enrollee, 1967–1986

Year	Enrollees (millions)	Reimbursement ($ billions)	Reimbursement per Enrollee ($)
1967	19.5	4.5	233
1968	19.8	5.7	287
1969	20.1	6.6	328
1970	20.5	7.1	346
1971	20.9	7.9	376
1972	21.3	8.6	405
1973	23.5	9.6	407
1974	24.2	12.4	513
1975	25.0	15.6	625
1976	25.7	18.4	718
1977	26.5	21.8	823
1978	27.2	24.9	918
1979	27.9	29.3	1053
1980	28.5	35.7	1253
1981	29.0	43.4	1497
1982	29.5	51.1	1732
1983	30.0	57.4	1913
1984	30.5	64.4	2111
1985	31.1	72.3	2249
1986	31.8	77.7	2443

Sources: Davis and Rowland 1986; 1988 unpublished Medicare statistics.

Medicare's Hospital Payment Policy

During legislative consideration of the Medicare program and its early enactment, the desire to accommodate the financial demands of hospitals, physicians, and other health care providers was a driving force in the formulation of Medicare payment policy. The fear that physicians and hospitals would boycott the new program led to many compromises (Feder 1977; Marmor 1973), one of which was the decision to use cost-based reimbursement methods for hospitals.

The legislation enacted by Congress gave the secretary of the Department of Health, Education, and Welfare (in 1980 renamed the Department of Health and Human Services [DHHS]) the authority to establish through the regulatory process the methods to be used to determine "reasonable costs" for purposes of reimbursing hospitals. The statute emphasized that the methods adopted should be based on consideration of principles already being used by national organizations (Feder 1977). In particular, the legislation followed the Blue Cross method of paying hospitals according to their costs.

The subsequent regulations, published by Medicare, affirmed the program's commitment to retrospective, cost-based reimbursement. Hospitals were to receive payment for any reasonable and necessary costs associated with the care of a patient (Feder 1977). In the early years hospitals also received an additional "2 percent plus" factor to encourage participation. Hospitals were assured retrospective reimbursement of the full costs of caring for Medicare beneficiaries, including the direct costs associated with each patient's care, such as room and board, as well as any ancillary service costs, such as diagnostic tests, surgical costs, and supplies. Medicare also reimbursed hospitals for the portion of overhead costs attributable to Medicare patients; these include administrative costs, utilities, rent, and other shared expenses. In addition, hospitals were paid for the portion of their capital costs attributable to their share of Medicare patients, including depreciation, interest expenses, rent, and the costs associated with training residents, nurses, and allied health professionals in teaching hospitals.

Under this reimbursement system, hospitals essentially were reimbursed for the cost of caring for a Medicare patient. Consequently, they had little financial incentive to operate efficiently. The greater an institution's costs, the greater would be its Medicare reimbursement. Basing hospital payments on cost, or cost-plus, was like giving hospitals a blank check to determine their own rate of payment. Soon after enactment, rising hospital expenditures raised concerns that the early principles were too favorable to the hospital industry (Weiner 1977). The 2 percent cost-plus factor was quickly dropped. Cost-based reimbursement continued, with Medicare paying a hospital its share of the hospital's operating expenses at the end of each year. The more a hospital spent, the more dollars it received from Medicare. There continued to be little incentive to be efficient or to restrain spending (Altman and Eichenholz 1976).

Under the Medicare legislation passed by Congress in 1965, the government was permitted to contract with fiscal intermediaries to administer the program and process claims (Starr 1982). In theory, by designating intermediaries to act as agents, the federal government was adhering to the principle of not interfering with the practice of medicine. However, the result was the creation of a third party, typically a Blue Cross plan with close ties to the hospital industry, to act on behalf of the federal government. This decision prevented federal officials from scrutinizing lengths of stay, admission rates, or the use of specific diagnostic tests, thereby severely limiting the ability to control costs.

Throughout the late 1960s the debate on reforming Medicare and the rising cost of care continued. Congress considered modifying the Medicare reimbursement system throughout this period. Feder reviewed the politics of the initial years of the Medicare program and concluded that "over the years of legislative consideration, government officials believed that a consensus had been reached on payment procedures, and they promised to follow established industry practices. But after enactment, the consensus disappeared as hospitals sought to acquire the most favorable payment arrangements they could" (Feder 1977).

The Economic Stabilization Program, 1972–1974

The Vietnam conflict left many legacies in the United States. President Johnson, unwilling to admit the full extent of early U.S. involvement, financed the war effort with federal budget deficits. This fiscal policy led to serious inflation in the late 1960s. Thus, incoming President Richard Nixon had to find solutions to thorny military and economic problems. In August 1971 President Nixon put a freeze on wages and prices in the entire economy, including the hospital industry, as part of his Economic Stabilization Program (ESP). During the period 1967–70, when the overall inflation in the economy was 5.2 percent, Medicare hospital expenditures increased at an annualized rate of 18.1 percent (HCFA 1987b). Health care costs were a source of special concern.

The freeze instituted in August 1971 was the first phase of ESP; it was replaced in December 1971 with phase 2, which comprised specific inflation targets for each major sector of the economy. The administration took more time to develop regulations for the health care sector than for other industries: regulations specific to hospitals were not issued until December 1972. The December 1972 regulations imposed a ceiling of 6 percent on price increases and required that all price increases be cost-justified. Limitations on specific cost increases were 5.5 percent for wages, 2.5 percent for nonlabor costs, and 1.7 percent for new technology and services.

By the time the health care industry regulations were finally promulgated, ESP had already begun lifting constraints on an industry-by-industry basis. Among the sectors remaining under control when ESP finally expired in April 1974 was the hospital sector. The president had implemented the program through an executive order; therefore, continuation of ESP for the health sector required legislation. When Congress sought to continue the controls established by ESP, the legislation was defeated because of strenuous opposition by the hospital industry.

The termination of controls on hospital expenditures during ESP cannot be attributed to lack of effectiveness. An initial review of the program using national data on hospital cost and revenue increases during the period from 1950–75 showed that the rate of increase in hospital room and board expenses had declined by 50 percent and that rates of increase in expenditures per diem and per admission had declined by 25 percent under ESP (Altman and Eichenholz 1976). Later, more sophisticated statistical studies showed annual reductions in the rate of increase in hospital expenditures due to ESP that varied between zero (Ginsburg 1978) and 2–3 percent (Sloan 1981). In a review of all the studies that investigated ESP, Steinwald and Sloan (1981) concluded: "Our summary statement, based upon both the descriptive and multivariate evidence, is that ESP did have a moderating influence on hospital cost inflation."

Once ESP controls were lifted, Medicare hospital expenditures increased even faster than they had prior to the imposition of controls. Clearly, temporary restraints had not cured the underlying inflation inherent in the hospital sector. The ESP and post-ESP periods demonstrated that long-term measures were required to control health care cost inflation.

The ESP controls on hospitals had an impact, however, beyond their immediate effect on hospital cost inflation. The ESP program's major effect was to demonstrate that across-the-board, all-payer rate-of-increase controls on hospital costs can be effective. ESP provides a concrete example of regulatory control on hospital costs that future regulators would draw upon. It is important to note also that the termination of ESP controls was based on the hospital industry's promise to restrain costs voluntarily. The inability of hospitals to do so set the stage for mandatory legislation in later years.

The Post–Economic Stabilization Program, 1975–1977

The period following the lifting of ESP controls on the hospital sector was marked by extremely rapid increases in health care costs. Nevertheless, several important cost containment initiatives were implemented during this period. Many of these initiatives were included in legislation passed by Congress in 1972 amending the original Medicare legislation. These amendments attempted to control both utilization of hospital services and Medicare hospital outlays. The regulations to implement this legislation were promulgated in 1975 and revised regularly during the period. A discussion of the amendments follows.

Section 223

Section 223 of the 1972 Medicare amendments gave Medicare the authority to disallow any costs unnecessary to the efficient provision of care. Since Medicaid hospital payment policy was tied to Medicare's, this provision extended to Medicaid as well. The amendment represented a major change in hospital payment policy. Prior to the passage of Section 223, Medicare's cost-based reimbursement policy had placed no constraints on allowable costs. As a result, cost increases were uncontrollable, and costs among hospitals for similar services varied considerably. The wide variation in costs per day at several hospitals captured the attention of Congress, which approved legislation aimed at eliminating this problem.

The purpose of Section 223 was to provide Medicare (and Medicaid, since states were required to follow Medicare hospital payment methods) with a means to deny payment to hospitals for costs that seemed unreasonably high in comparison with those of other hospitals. The original methodology for determining excessive costs was quite crude; as a result, DHHS chose to set the limits sufficiently high that few hospitals would be affected. As the methodology was refined and additional cost savings were desired, the 223 limits were gradually lowered to affect more hospitals. The 223 limits never generated significant cost savings, but they are important because they laid the groundwork for controlling hospital costs and eventually formed the basis for methodologies used in the Medicare Prospective Payment System.

When Section 223 regulations limiting allowable costs were first implemented on July 1, 1974, they applied only to routine costs and did not include ancillary services, special care units, or outpatient care. A hospital's routine costs include room, board, and nursing costs. Routine cost per day, rather than total costs per admission, was selected as the basis for limits. The reason for this lay in the fact that total cost per admission is much more sensitive to the hospital's case mix. For example, the average length of stay in a hospital that treats patients with more complex illnesses will be longer than that in a hospital that treats patients with less complex illnesses. Similarly, the cost of ancillary services will be greater in the former. On the other hand, "hotel" costs, food costs, and nursing care per day should be roughly the same.

Several calculations were made in order to establish limits on allowable costs. Adjustments were necessary to reflect factors that could affect routine cost per day. Hospitals were grouped according to hospital bed size and location (rural or urban). In addition, hospital costs were adjusted for the per capita income of the community in which the hospital was located. This adjustment served as a proxy for differences in wages of hospital personnel and other input costs. Costs were projected for the coming year using estimates of hospital cost increases developed by Medicare actuaries. Ceilings on maximum allowable payment were determined by ranking hospitals from lowest to highest cost per day and then determining a certain cutoff value to be the maximum reimbursable cost limit.

It was generally recognized that these methods were relatively crude and needed to be refined. Economists and other social scientists had begun to conduct research on hospital cost functions but had not reached a consensus on the factors that significantly influenced hospital costs. Most of the early analyses showed that hospital bed size, geographic location, and some measure of input costs were important predictors of hospital costs (Carr and Feldstein 1967; Lave, Lave, and Silverman 1972).

Probably the most important determinant of the method used by DHHS, however, was the availability of data that could be useful in establishing limits. For example, there were no suitable case mix measures to quantify the output of hospitals (Sloan, Feldman, and Steinwald 1983). For this reason, ancillary costs, which are not the same for all medical problems, were not included in the calculation. A desire to expand the 223 limits to cover total costs per admission was a major impetus for research on case mix measures that led to the DRG system (Pettingill and Vertrees 1982).

Promulgation of regulations establishing the original limits and their subsequent application to specific hospitals led to many refinements in the 223 methodology. The original proxy for input costs—per capita income in the county—was soon replaced by a wage index for hospital workers. The wage index compared the hourly wage for nonsupervisory hospital workers in each standard metropolitan statistical area (SMSA) with the national average. Similar indexes for the rural part of each state were created. Eventually the actuarial projections of hospital costs were replaced by a hospital input price index using an econometric model to project the rate of increase in hospital production costs (Freeland, Anderson, and Schendler 1979). The hospital market basket, a measure of the inflation rate in inputs purchased by hospitals, was created when hospitals became concerned that the federal government would lower the inflation projection to generate budgetary savings. The actual 1980 Section 223 limits for hospitals are shown in table 2.2.

As the Section 223 limits became more stringent, hospital administrators and federal policymakers became interested in examining which hospitals were being affected by them. Because the limits did not initially recognize the costs associated with operating an educational program, teaching hospitals were found to be disproportionately penalized. Eventually they were permitted to exclude direct teaching costs from their allowable costs before determining whether their allowable costs were below the limits. These costs included the salaries and fringe benefits of residents, teaching physicians, and other instructors, as well as the administrative costs of operating an educational program.

Even when direct teaching costs were excluded from the calculation, teaching hospitals were more likely than nonteaching hospitals to reach

Table 2.2. Section 223 Limits on Allowable Costs per Day for Seven Hospital Categories, 1980

Category	Cost per Day	Category	Cost per Day
Urban		Rural	
Fewer than 100 beds	$128.72	Fewer than 100 beds	119.32
101 to 404 beds	128.53	100 to 169 beds	119.15
405 to 684 beds	124.34	170 beds or more	115.14
685 beds or more	131.48		

Source: DHHS 1980.

or exceed 223 limits on costs per day. In 1980 the concept of indirect teaching costs was developed. The indirect teaching adjustment is a proxy for costs experienced by teaching hospitals that cannot be measured directly. The level of adjustment is determined by comparing the costs of teaching and nonteaching hospitals, controlling for other factors such as bed size and input costs, and calculating the factor necessary to ensure that the same percentage of teaching and nonteaching hospitals is affected by the 223 limits. In other words, the adjustment for indirect costs is based on the assumption that teaching and nonteaching hospitals are equally efficient and that the indirect costs associated with teaching are legitimate costs (Anderson and Lave 1986). This assumption of a "level playing field" is a common theme of most hospital payment reforms.

In the evolution of hospital payment, 223 limits are important for three reasons. First, they demonstrate Congress's concern over increasing hospital costs in the Medicare program and its willingness to tighten the "reasonable cost" definition. Enactment of 223 is also evidence of Congress's willingness to implement Medicare controls while rejecting the across-the-board controls of ESP. With Section 223, hospitals were put on notice that some test of efficiency would be applied to their Medicare costs, thus limiting the original blank-check approach. Second, authority to limit reimbursement under 223 gave the administration a regulatory tool to use in restraining costs under Medicare. This was increasingly important in the late 1970s as pressure increased to restrain Medicare's growing hospital payments. Third, the 223 regulations led to the development of methodology and data sources that were important to the development of future payment reform.

Professional Standards Review Organizations

The 1972 Medicare amendments created the Professional Standards Review Organizations (PSROs) to monitor the quality of federally funded care and to ensure its delivery in the most efficient and economical man-

Table 2.3. Medicare Hospital Utilization, 1967–1986

Year	Inpatient Days (millions)	Percentage Increase from Previous Years
1967	70	
1968	75	7.5
1969	77	2.1
1970	76	−0.7
1971	75	−1.6
1972	76	1.2
1973	79	4.1
1974	87	9.0
1975	90	2.6
1976	95	5.0
1977	96	1.4
1978	98	2.1
1979	101	2.4
1980	107	6.1
1981	109	1.6
1982	114	4.5
1983	116	1.7
1984	105	−10.0
1985	94	−12.0
1986	91	−3.0

Source: HCFA 1988 unpublished data.

ner. PSROs were created in response to increases in Medicare utilization rates not anticipated by the drafters of the legislation. During the period 1967–72 the number of inpatient days increased at an annual rate of 1.8 percent (see table 2.3).

Prior to the 1970s, utilization review was performed by individual hospitals using internal review panels to monitor the technical quality of care and the necessity of services prescribed. These activities were a requirement for participation in the Medicare program from its inception. Every participating hospital had to establish utilization review panels to review the necessity of each admission, length of stay, and specific services delivered. For example, patients with extended stays were required to be recertified at periodic intervals in order to establish the necessity for continued hospital care. These programs generally emulated the Blue Cross utilization review programs already in operation.

The 1972 amendments designated 203 local areas in which PSROs would be established to review the appropriateness of care provided to all Medicare, Medicaid, and Maternal and Child Health patients. PSRO areas could be as large as an entire state or as small as a few zip code areas within a single city. PSROs were federally funded, but they relied upon locally developed standards.

One of the program's many objectives was to monitor admissions and lengths of stay of hospitalized patients. The data generated by this function demonstrated that there was considerable variation in medical practices in different regions of the country. Days of care per 1,000 Medicare enrollees in 1974 varied from 2,023 in the Fresno-Madera area of California to 5,283 in the Adirondack region of New York (Deacon et al. 1979). Similar variations in admission rates and average lengths of stay were discovered by other researchers (Wennberg 1984). One of the major methodological developments of the PSRO program was the creation of diagnosis-related groups (DRGs), which were used to group patients with similar lengths of stay. These classifications were developed to help PSROs monitor the average length of stay of hospitalized patients.

Although it was generally agreed that the objectives of the PSRO program were important, a number of legislative and regulatory restrictions made it difficult for the program to achieve its goals. First, the statute mandated that only physicians were permitted to review the treatment of hospitalized Medicare beneficiaries. Many physicians were reluctant to monitor the care provided by other physicians, so the review process was more lax than its creators had intended.

A second problem was that the emphasis on local medical practice made it nearly impossible to eliminate regional variations in practice patterns or to establish nationally acceptable standards for admission or length of stay. Empirical studies showed that utilization rates and expenditures per Medicare beneficiary in one PSRO area could be double the rates in another (Deacon et al. 1979; Gornick, Newton, and Hackerman 1980).

A third problem was that although hospitals could be denied payment when an admission or extra days of care were deemed inappropriate, physician payments were not constrained. This policy created a conflict, because a hospital was liable for the actions of its admitting physicians, who had little incentive to curtail patient hospital use. It is not surprising that some evaluations of the program showed it to be marginally cost-effective (Dobson et al. 1978), while others demonstrated that the government spent more funds to operate the program than it saved through lower utilization rates (CBO 1979b, 1981).

Section 1122

Section 1122 authorized state-designated planning agencies to review hospital plans for expansion and modernization. Capital projects that were not approved were not eligible for capital reimbursement by the

Medicare, Medicaid, or Maternal and Child Health programs, although the hospital could try to secure funds from other third-party payers to over costs.

The 1122 process was strengthened with the passage of Public Law 93-641, the National Health Planning and Resource Development Act of 1974 (Altman, Greene, and Sapolsky 1981; Lefkowitz 1983). This law created a network of health planning agencies that monitored the allocation of health facilities in each geographic area. The health planning agencies were to review local needs and make recommendations to state planning agencies regarding approval or denial of Certificate of Need (CON) applications.

Designated planning agencies were to receive federal funds to perform this function and were to use national criteria to monitor projects. Initially, any projects that changed bed capacity or service capacity or had costs exceeding $100,000 were required to obtain CON approval. These conditions were changed as the program evolved.

Most of the empirical research on 1122 and CON reviews suggests that they have been only marginally successful in controlling per diem, per admission, or per capita costs. Studies generally conclude that although these programs may have controlled the number of beds to some extent, hospitals have responded to the controls by adding more equipment or other capital assets per bed. Salkever and Bice (1979) found that state CON controls had no effect on total capital assets but may have caused some hospitals to substitute equipment for beds.

The limited impact of the CON and health planning process on health care costs is not surprising given the absence of any effective sanctions or incentives for local or state planning agencies to disapprove CON applications. No caps were placed on the total volume of projects that could be approved. Planning agencies, therefore, were not forced to make real choices among alternatives. Approval of projects resulted in more services to the community and more jobs, both of which appealed to consumer-dominated boards. The fiscal consequences of approving capital expansions were diffused broadly to taxpayers and employers as the Medicare, Medicaid, and private insurance plans paid the cost indirectly through outlays for patient care.

Section 222 and State Cost Containment Efforts

The 1972 amendments implicitly acknowledged that effective methods of stopping the extraordinary rise in hospital expenditures were not known, yet the current system needed revision. Therefore, they encouraged experimentation with innovative payment demonstrations. Section 222 of the amendments supported incentive reimbursement demonstrations, voluntary and mandatory rate-setting programs, alternative care demonstrations (e.g., ambulatory surgery), and a wide variety of innovative approaches to health care cost containment.

This provision helped stimulate and assist several states to develop their own approaches to cost containment, primarily through the establishment of state rate-setting agencies. By 1976 six states (Connecticut, Maryland, Massachusetts, New Jersey, New York, and Washington) had enacted mandatory rate regulation programs and had proceeded to regulate hospitals (Biles, Schramm, and Atkinson 1980). Unique political forces in each state lay behind the legislated approach taken; however, all six states shared certain characteristics. In general, they had higher hospital costs per admission than other states. They had relatively generous Medicaid programs, representing significant state fiscal outlays. Finally, Blue Cross had a significant market share.

State programs to control costs varied considerably in terms of the administrative body responsible for the program, the extent of controls (mandatory or voluntary), payers covered (Medicare, Medicaid, or private health insurance), program methodology (budget review, formula, etc.), method of control (total revenues, revenue per case, cost-based limit on charges, etc.) and unit of payment (charges, per diem, cost per case, or annual percentage of total budget) (Bauer 1977).

In addition to the fully mandatory approach, some states developed more limited voluntary approaches to cost control, often in cooperation with Blue Cross or, sometimes, the state hospital association. In addition to the six states with mandatory programs cited above, approximately ten states had implemented voluntary programs as of May 1982 (Esposito et al. 1982).

Most of the evidence shows the mandatory state rate-setting programs to be an effective means of constraining hospital costs. A comparison of the expenses per admission in the six rate-setting states with those in the forty-four nonregulated states during the period 1975–78 shows that rate-setting states restrained the rate of increase in hospital costs to 11.2 percent, while the rate increase in states without programs was 14.3 percent (Biles, Schramm, and Atkinson 1980). This study was confirmed by numerous econometric analyses that found significant evidence of substantial reductions in hospital rate of growth in mature rate-setting programs (CBO 1979a; Coelen and Sullivan 1981; Steinwald and Sloan 1981).

The state experience with rate setting was a critical factor in the evolution of hospital payment policy at the federal level. The state experience demonstrated that a regulatory approach works, and works well, to restrain hospital costs. The states were a testing site for the prospective rate-setting approach and helped to refine and improve the methodology for rate setting and prospective payment. New Jersey pioneered the DRG system later adopted by the Medicare program (Iglehart 1982c).

Other Federal Efforts to Shape the Health Care System

The early 1970s saw several major pieces of federal legislation designed to shape the future direction of the health care system. The increase in health care costs following the introduction of Medicare and Medicaid led to a policy of expanding supply to control costs (DHEW 1971). This policy is based on the economic principle that an increase in supply will result in a decline in price. The Emergency Health Personnel Act of 1970 created the National Health Service Corps to provide physicians and other health professionals to underserved areas. The Health Manpower Training Act of 1970 further encouraged the training of physicians but put new emphasis on training primary care physicians (rather than specialists). The Health Maintenance Organization Act of 1973 established a federal grant and loan program to encourage the development of HMOs and required employers to offer employees the choice of enrolling in an HMO.

The Carter Hospital Cost Containment Bill and the Hospital Industry Voluntary Effort, 1978–1980

When President Carter assumed office in January 1977, hospital expenses were increasing rapidly. Community hospital expenses in 1975, 1976, and 1977 had increased at an average annual rate that was 8.7 percent higher than the overall inflation rate (AHA 1986). This increase posed a serious obstacle to two presidential objectives: balancing the federal budget and enacting a national health plan to expand health insurance coverage to the entire population.

In February 1977 the president announced his intention to submit a major legislative proposal constraining the rate of increases in hospital costs. The issue of rising costs and attempts to contain hospital inflation came to dominate the health policy agenda throughout the Carter administration. The Carter bill was based on an across-the-board, all-payer approach to hospital cost containment. For a variety of reasons it never was enacted into law.

The First Round

In April 1977 President Carter forwarded to Congress a legislative proposal to limit the rate of increase in hospital revenues (H.R. 6575). This bill proposed to limit the rate of increase in hospital revenues for all patients to about 3 percent over the overall inflation rate (as measured by the Gross National Product price deflator). The bill had several features:

- It applied to all patients and was enforced through separate limits on the rate of increase in revenues from Medicare, Medicaid, Blue Cross, and all other payers.
- It exempted states with mandatory, all-payer hospital rate-setting programs.
- It gave hospitals an incentive to reduce the number of admissions.
- It proposed limits on total hospital capital investment in order to strengthen CON and health planning laws and to induce planning agencies to set priorities among alternative projects.

The proposal was presented as an interim measure while a longer-term prospective payment system was developed (Califano 1977). It was estimated that the bill would reduce the federal budget by approximately $20 billion over a five-year period and reduce private health insurance outlays by another $30 billion over the same period.

The bill was opposed vigorously by both the hospital industry and the medical profession. Enormous political pressure to oppose this legislation was placed on key congressional members (Abernethy and Pearson 1979). Campaign contributions from hospital and medical interest groups were highly correlated with votes against the bill. Fragmentation of congressional jurisdiction led to lengthy delays in enactment. The legislation came under the jurisdiction of four different committees, two in the House and two in the Senate, each with its own health subcommittee. To be approved, the bill needed to win approval in all subcommittees, all four full committees, and on the floor of the House and Senate.

Analytical arguments presented by the industry were also a factor in building opposition to the bill:

- The bill provided no reward for efficiency. Hospitals with high costs would get the same percentage rate of increase as hospitals with low costs.
- The bill did not recognize the diversity of American hospitals and thus did not take into account the special problems of individual hospitals.
- The GNP price deflator did not appropriately reflect the inflation in prices of goods and services purchased by hospitals, such as malpractice insurance and electricity.
- The cap on capital investment and the limit on hospital revenues would discourage innovation, improvements in technology, and quality of care.

The most persuasive argument put forth by the hospital industry, however, was that voluntary efforts on the part of hospitals would contain costs without federal legislation. Congressman Dan Rostenkowski (D-Ill.), chairman of the House Ways and Means Committee Subcommittee on Health, challenged the hospital industry to control hospital costs voluntarily. He proposed that Congress approve legislation imposing mandatory limits only if voluntary efforts failed, and he spearheaded passage of a bill with this modification through the subcommittee.

The hospital industry responded by forming the Voluntary Effort (VE), a coalition of providers and payers, in December 1977. The VE established national and state goals to reduce the rate of increase in hospital costs by 2 percent annually in 1978 and 1979 relative to the 1977 rate of increase. Other goals were established for increases in hospital beds, employees per patient, and capital investment (see table 2.4). The hospital industry succeeded in reaching its target for 1978, despite accelerated inflation in the economy as a whole.

In the closing days of the 95th Congress the Senate passed a modified version of the Carter bill sponsored by Senator Nelson (D-Wis.). This bill included a trigger that would introduce mandatory limits only if voluntary efforts to limit increases in hospital costs did not succeed. Both major subcommittees with jurisdiction over the bill, the House Subcommittee on Health and the Environment and the House Ways and Means Health Subcommittee, had approved versions. However, time ran out, and the 95th Congress expired without action being taken by the full House.

Round Two

During the 96th Congress the Carter administration reviewed the analytical arguments against its cost containment bill and modified it substantially. In March 1979 the administration introduced a new hospital cost containment bill, H.R. 2626, in the 96th Congress. The new bill addressed many of the concerns raised by the hospital industry and congressional leaders:

- It contained a voluntary trigger, specifying that mandatory limits would only be imposed on any given hospital if national, state, and individual hospital voluntary limits were not met. The voluntary limits were approximately the same as the goals of the VE group.

- The mandatory limit on total revenues was set at the projected increase in the hospital market basket price index, plus 1 percent, plus an allowance for population growth. Using a hospital market basket price index instead of the GNP price deflator guaranteed hospitals an increase adequate to cover inflation in the costs of goods and services they actually purchased.

- The 1 percent additional allowance provided an explicit allowance for new technology and improvements in quality.

Table 2.4. **Voluntary Effort Targets Set by the Hospital Industry Compared with Actual Performance, 1979–1981**

Year	Goal	Actual Performance
	Annual Increase in Hospital Expenses (%)	
1978	13.6	12.8
1979	11.6	13.4
1980	11.9	16.8
1981	less than 6.8	17.8
	Annual Increase in Beds (no.)	
1978	0	10,289
1979	0	13,481
1980	−3,192	16,827
1981	0	9,307
	Annual Increase in Employees per Patient Census (%)	
1978	1.6	3.1
1979	−0.4	1.8
1980	less than 1.8	1.2
1981	less than 1.2	1.7
	Annual Increase in Capital ($ billions)	
1978	3.15	3.24
1979	3.01	3.64
1980	—	—
1981	—	—

- Rewards for efficiency were built in. Hospitals received a higher or lower rate of increase revenue limit depending upon whether their routine costs per day were above or below the average for similar hospitals (using the Section 223 methodology).

- Certain hospitals were exempted from the limits. These included small, rural hospitals, children's hospitals, and regional tertiary care institutions.

- States with mandatory all-payer rate-setting programs were exempt.

- The limit on capital investment was omitted.

- A sunset clause required that the law expire after five years and be replaced by a permanent prospective payment system. A commission was to be established to develop such a system.

Table 2.5. Estimated Impact of the Mandatory Provisions of the Carter Hospital Cost Containment Bill of 1979 (H.R. 2626)

Fiscal Year	Federal Budget Savings ($ millions)	Total System Savings ($ millions)	Increase in Hospital Costs (%)	
			Without bill	With bill
1980	1,120	2,900	13.0	8.9
1981	2,470	6,320	13.9	9.1
1982	3,970	9,970	14.0	10.0
1983	5,690	14,050	13.1	9.5
1984	7,630	18,530	11.7	8.3
Total	20,880	51,770	13.1[a]	9.2[a]

Source: HCFA, Division of Medicare Cost Estimates, unpublished data, 15 May 1979.
[a]Average over 1980–84 period.

The new bill also was projected to achieve considerable federal budgetary savings and savings to the private health insurance sector. As shown in table 2.5, it was estimated that the net effect of the bill would be to lower the rate of increase in hospital costs by about 3–4 percent a year below what would have otherwise occurred. The total savings to the federal budget over the period 1980–84 was estimated to be $21 billion; the total system savings, including savings to both the public and the private sector, was estimated to be $52 billion over the five-year period.

Between March and November 1979 the bill was passed with modifications by three major committees: the House Ways and Means Committee, the House Energy and Commerce Committee, and the Senate Human Resources Committee. Under the various versions savings to the total system over five years ranged from $30 billion to $50 billion.

The hospital industry continued to oppose mandatory legislation. It argued that the modifications—made in response to hospital industry complaints about the 1977 bill—were now too complex and would prove difficult to administer. In addition, the hospital industry pointed to the major slowdown in hospital cost increases in 1978 and 1979, years when inflation in the economy was reaching double-digit rates because of OPEC oil price hikes. The legislation was defeated on the floor of the House in November 1979, and efforts to obtain a mandatory law controlling hospital costs for all patients ceased.

Despite the legislative defeat, the hospital cost containment initiative is critical to the evolution and understanding of federal hospital payment policy. First, it brought the issue of rising hospital costs and the need to address them to the attention of Congress and the American people. The issue was not whether costs for hospital care were too high but whether the industry could voluntarily bring costs down without federal regulation. Congress elected to try the voluntary approach. Just as in 1974, when the hospital industry defeated extension of across-the-board controls under ESP phase 4 on the grounds that it could voluntarily curb hospital rates, in 1979 the hospital industry again argued that it would get its own house in order and was again successful in resisting regulation. This assurance of cost restraint by the industry in 1979 and the industry's subsequent failure helped lay the groundwork for the changes in hospital payment enacted in 1982.

The major difference between the Carter hospital cost containment legislation and subsequent legislative proposals was its all-payer approach. The Carter administration argued that a Medicare-only system would discriminate against elderly patients, leading to a two-class system of care. They also argued that the hospital cost problem was systemic and thus required systemwide solutions for both public and private patients.

The Voluntary Effort

The VE figured importantly in the defeat of the Carter hospital cost containment legislation. The VE was a coalition of health care provider organizations (most notably the AHA, the Federation of American Hospitals, the AMA, and Blue Cross/Blue Shield). The VE provided a private-sector alternative to federal regulation of hospital costs. It included state-level cost containment committees to "jawbone" the industry. National target rates of increase were proposed for 1978 and 1979 to try to restrain cost increases.

During consideration of the cost containment legislation in 1978 the VE was able to obtain its goal, and hospitals successfully held down the rate of increase despite a rapid acceleration in economywide inflation caused by an increase in oil prices. Initially the Congressional Budget Office found that the VE had a small, negative impact on hospital expenditure increases (CBO 1979a). Sloan found that while the VE helped reduce costs per adjusted admission and per patient day, at the same time it also contributed to an increase in profits (Steinwald and Sloan 1981). These positive findings were short-lived, however; as soon as the threat of regulation was removed in 1979, hospital costs began to climb once more, and the VE ended almost immediately (Davis 1981).

Section 223 Limits

During consideration of hospital cost containment and especially in the wake of the defeat of the legislation, limits on Medicare reimbursement for hospital care under Section 223 resurfaced as part of the federal hospital payment strategy. Tightening the 223 limits did not require new legislation but could be accomplished by regulatory change under existing authority. Thus, when the hospital cost containment legislation stalled in Congress, the administration turned to Medicare 223 limits as a way to achieve some of the savings desired in the federal budget. It should be noted that although the administration favored and sought all-payer, across-the-board hospital cost regulation, the pressures of the budget resulted in use of the Medicare-only 223 limit approach as a fallback. While the 223 methodology was refined and the limits were tightened, it never achieved the savings proposed in the cost containment legislation.

A desire to broaden the scope of 223 limits in order to cover more than routine costs per day led to the development of total cost limits that included the limits on the costs of ancillary services. Research on DRGs was conducted at Yale University, tested in the New Jersey rate-setting demonstration, and studied within DHHS. This helped lay the groundwork for the next generation of cost containment proposals, the prospective payment DRG system.

Major Lessons

Consideration of the Carter hospital cost containment legislation represented a major political struggle over a three-year period with several significant outcomes. First, it slowed the rate of increase in hospital costs over the term of the Carter presidency. The rate of increase in community hospital expenses (deflated by the Consumer Price Index) fell from 9.5 percent in 1976, when President Carter took office, to 1.7 percent in 1979, at the height of the debate over legislation, and was at 2.6 percent in 1980, when he left office. Statistical studies confirmed the deflationary effect of the Carter hospital cost containment bill and the hospital industry response in the form of the VE.

Second, the Carter bill was extremely important in setting the political groundwork for successful passage of Medicare hospital payment reform in 1982 and 1983. It raised general public awareness of the problem of rising hospital costs; it informed key congressional leaders about the problem; and most important, the disillusionment with the hospital industry's broken promise to constrain costs voluntarily led to widespread bipartisan support for major changes in Medicare hospital payment policies in 1982 and 1983.

Finally, the Carter administration sponsored the analytic work and data base development that permitted the development of the DRG prospective payment proposal adopted in 1983. In his testimony before the Senate Finance Committee in 1977 Secretary of Health and Human Services Joseph A. Califano pledged to develop the data and methodology necessary to implement a prospective payment system based on patient case mix (Califano 1977). The Carter bill in 1979 already reflected progress in this direction with the development of a hospital market basket index, a refined Section 223 methodology for measuring and encouraging hospital efficiency, and a proposal for a commission to develop a long-term prospective payment system. Under Section 223 authority, DHHS supported state experiments with prospective payment systems, including the DRG all-payer prospective payment system in New Jersey. The experience and methodological tools that would be required to design and implement a prospective payment system were underway.

Chapter 3   The Reagan Administration and
              Medicare Hospital Payment

Reforming the health care system and changing the method of paying for hospital services was not an early priority of the Reagan administration. However, when hospital costs began increasing rapidly in the Medicare program shortly after President Reagan took office, a team of analysts from both within and outside the federal government began developing policy options for controlling hospital costs. The advisors decided that cost containment could be achieved through competition and deregulation. The Reagan administration announced its intention to develop legislation to promote competition in the health sector as a means of curbing costs, but internal dissension and congressional skepticism caused those proposals to be left on the drawing board. Instead, a more pragmatic approach developed.

Congressional Action to Limit Hospital Medicare and Medicaid Hospital Payments, 1981

Rapid increases in health care costs and in government outlays for Medicare and Medicaid characterized the early 1980s under the Reagan administration. Congress soon insisted that changes be made in Medicare and Medicaid to limit payments. Congressional action was driven in large part by a desire to find an alternative to Reagan administration proposals to cut the benefit and eligibility standards in the Medicare and Medicaid programs. Congress worked to substitute cuts that would fall on providers rather than on beneficiaries.

The Omnibus Budget Reconciliation Act of 1981 (OBRA) made only minor changes in the Medicare program. The limits on Medicare reimbursement under Section 223 were tightened legislatively to generate additional savings. The Secretary of Health and Human Services was required to develop a new system for hospital services under Medicare and Medicaid and to report to Congress on this system by July 1982. The

Table 3.1. Projected TEFRA Savings, 1983–1985

Fiscal Year	Savings ($ millions)
1983	480
1984	1,770
1985	3,770
Total	6,020

Source: Congress 1982.

major change was that states were given flexibility to design and implement their own hospital payment plans for Medicaid. This led to a number of Medicaid-only prospective payment systems in subsequent years.

The Tax Equity and Fiscal Responsibility Act of 1982

The Tax Equity and Fiscal Responsibility Act of 1982 (TEFRA) mandated significant changes in hospital payment rates directed primarily at controlling the rate of growth in Medicare hospital expenditures (Iglehart 1982b). It was the first major action by Congress aimed at controlling hospital spending. Three features of the TEFRA system were of particular importance.

First, it established a limit on the rate of increase over time in Medicare hospital payment rates. Medicare payments per admission were constrained to increase no faster than the rate of increase in the hospital market basket plus an allowance of 1 percent for new technology and services (Freeland, Anderson, and Schendler 1979). If hospital costs increased less than this amount, a hospital was paid its costs; if cost increases were greater than this amount, Medicare payment was limited to this rate of increase. The 1 percent allowance for new technology and services was lower than the historical rate of 2.3 percent (1974–82), placing a significant constraint on increases in Medicare payments (Anderson 1986).

Second, TEFRA modified the Section 223 limits to incorporate a case mix index based upon DRGs and provided incentive payments to hospitals defined as efficient. The tougher 223 limits, coupled with the rate-of-increase limit enacted in TEFRA, were to save $6 billion in Medicare hospital payments over three years (see table 3.1). Third, Congress directed the Department of Health and Human Services to develop by December 1982 a legislative proposal under which Medicare would pay hospitals prospectively.

The TEFRA system was initiated and developed by Congress. The driving force behind its passage was the desire to achieve budgetary savings in Medicare. The continued escalation of hospital costs, the concern over projected deficits in the Medicare trust funds, and the inability of the hospital industry to control costs voluntarily stimulated Congress to take action to control hospital expenditures.

TEFRA applied exclusively to hospital care received by Medicare beneficiaries, or about 35 percent of hospital total patient revenues. In contrast, the Nixon Economic Stabilization Program applied to all patients, as did the Carter hospital cost containment proposal. With TEFRA, Congress essentially passed the Carter cost containment legislation for Medicare only, thereby restricting health care cost containment efforts to the Medicare program. After 1981 state Medicaid programs were free to develop their own hospital payment methods and could choose to follow the Medicare prospective payment system or any other reasonable approach. Private health insurance plans were not addressed.

The Significance of TEFRA

The TEFRA system went into effect in October 1982 and was replaced by the Medicare Prospective Payment System (PPS) in October 1983. Although short-lived, TEFRA was significant in three respects. First and foremost, it achieved significant budgetary savings. The PPS legislation in 1983 was budget-neutral; that is, it did not attempt to achieve any budgetary savings over and beyond those contained in TEFRA. Second, PPS was phased in gradually, so that elements of the TEFRA system continued to affect hospitals up until 1988. Third, the TEFRA provisions introduced much of the conceptual and methodological features contained in the PPS legislation.

One major methodological development in TEFRA was the introduction of a case mix measure into the federal hospital payment formula. Previously, under Section 223, determination of hospital efficiency for the purpose of establishing limits on cost reimbursement was based on a comparison of hospital routine costs—the approximately 50 percent of hospital expenditures related to room and board, administration, and nursing services. Comparison was also restricted to per diem costs, because length of stay is related to a hospital's case mix. Without a case mix measure, a per-admission comparison is inappropriate. With the addition of a case mix measure, reasonable-cost limits could be established on the basis of total operating cost per patient discharge.

TEFRA mandated that limits on costs per discharge be set using the case mix measure developed at Yale University known as diagnosis-related groups (DRGs) (Fetter et al. 1977). This system classifies hospital inpatients into patient care categories according to the patient's primary and secondary diagnosis, procedures performed, age, discharge status, and whether the patient had certain complications and/or comorbidities. Using this system, diagnoses are first grouped into twenty-three major organ systems and then subdivided further so that patients within each group require similar levels of resources. A major assumption of the DRG system is that patients within each DRG are homogeneous with respect to their consumption of hospital resources. The number of groups changes periodically and is approaching five hundred. The first thirty-five DRGs, all of which pertain to diseases of the nervous system, are listed in table 3.2.

Medicare payment limits per discharge were calculated by comparing similar hospitals (based on the same bed size and geographic location categories used earlier for Section 223 limits) and adjusting for case mix differences (using the DRG case mix classification system), input prices, and teaching status (Vladeck 1984). Hospitals whose expenditures per discharge exceeded 112 percent of their peer group's average had their payment limit set at 112 percent of the group average. The percentage was scheduled to decline to 108 percent of the group average over the next three years. The specific level of 112 percent was chosen in order to generate the same budgetary savings as had been generated by the earlier 223 limits and because there was a perception that the methodology was too crude to tighten the limits any further.

Finally, TEFRA introduced into the Medicare payment system rewards for efficient performance. Under TEFRA the hospital had two constraints: a limit on the rate of increase in Medicare hospital payments per discharge (market basket plus 1 percent) and a peer group limit on the level of hospital expenses per discharge. If a hospital's actual expenditures were less than both of the limits, the hospital's incentive payment would be equal to one-half of the difference between the lower of the two limits and its actual costs. If a hospital's costs exceeded either or both of the limits, it would receive a payment equal to the lower of the two limits (Schweiker 1983).

In summary, TEFRA limited the rate of increase in hospital payments to a federally established rate, applied the program to Medicare patients exclusively, introduced the DRGs into the payment formula, permitted efficient hospitals to retain some of the savings, and penalized hospitals for inefficiency. TEFRA also borrowed many ideas from the Medicare Section 223 regulations, including separate limits for urban and rural hospitals, the wage index, and special adjustments for teaching hospitals (TEFRA 1982).

Flaws in TEFRA

Despite the advances TEFRA represented over the prior cost-based reimbursement system, it fell short of an ideal system in two major respects.

Table 3.2. **DRGs, DRG Weights, Lengths of Stay, and Outlier Thresholds in Major Diagnostic Category 1 (MDC1), Diseases of the Nervous System, 1986**

DRG	Title	DRG Weight	Mean Length of Stay	Outlier Threshold
1	Craniotomy except for trauma, age greater than 17	3.5632	16.2	33
2	Craniotomy for trauma, age greater than 17	3.8117	13.4	30
3	Craniotomy, age less than 18	2.9183	12.7	30
4	Spinal procedures	2.7300	15.0	32
5	Extracranial vascular procedures	1.6510	8.0	25
6	Carpal tunnel release	0.4072	2.3	7
7	Peripheral and cranial nerve, other nervous system procedures, age greater than 69, or comorbidity or complications	1.3867	6.1	23
8	Peripheral and cranial nerve, other nervous system procedures, age less than 70, without comorbidity or complications	0.7466	3.7	19
9	Spinal disorders and injuries	1.4237	8.4	25
10	Nervous system neoplasms, age greater than 69, or comorbidity or complications	1.1324	7.8	25
11	Nervous system neoplasms, age less than 70, without comorbidity or complications	0.9338	6.1	23
12	Degenerative nervous system disorders	1.0016	7.8	25
13	Multiple sclerosis and cerebellar ataxia	0.9789	7.7	25
14	Specific cerebrovascular disorders except TIA	1.3144	8.5	26
15	Transient ischemic attack and precerebral occlusions	0.6241	4.7	19
16	Nonspecific cerebrovascular disorders with comorbidity or complications	0.9044	6.8	24
17	Nonspecific cerebrovascular disorders without comorbidity or complications	0.6803	5.6	23
18	Cranial and peripheral nerve disorders, age greater than 60, or comorbidity or complications	0.7567	6.1	23

Table 3.2. Continued

DRG	Title	DRG Weight	Mean Length of Stay	Outlier Threshold
19	Cranial and peripheral nerve disorders, age less than 70, without comorbidity or complications	0.6548	5.3	22
20	Nervous system infection except viral meningitis	1.4090	7.8	25
21	Viral meningitis	1.3144	7.9	25
22	Hypertensive encephalopathy	0.7087	5.0	20
23	Nontraumatic stupor and coma	1.1242	5.2	22
24	Seizure and headache, age greater than 69, or comorbidity or complications	0.7644	5.0	22
25	Seizure and headache, age 18–69, without comorbidity or complications	0.5522	4.0	18
26	Seizure or headache, age less than 18	0.6255	2.7	14
27	Traumatic stupor and coma, coma greater than 1 hour	1.5648	4.7	22
28	Traumatic stupor and coma, coma less than 1 hour, age greater than 69, or comorbidity or complications	0.9422	5.0	22
29	Traumatic stupor and coma, less than 1 hour, age 18–69, without comorbidity or complications	0.6462	3.6	21
30	Traumatic stupor or coma, less than 1 hour, age less than 18	0.3539	2.0	8
31	Concussion, age greater than 69, or comorbidity or complications	0.5383	3.9	20
32	Concussion, age 18–69, without comorbidity or complications	0.4064	2.9	14
33	Concussion, age less than 18	0.2457	1.6	5
34	Other disorders of nervous system, age greater than 69, or comorbidity or complications	0.9777	6.1	23
35	Other disorders of nervous system, age less than 70, without comorbidity or complications	0.7384	4.9	22

Source: DHHS 1985.

First, it granted the same rate of increase to all hospitals, regardless of whether they had high or low costs initially. Thus, an inefficient hospital whose costs were twice as high as an efficient hospital would get the same increase as the efficient hospital. The absolute difference in Medicare payment to the two hospitals would widen over time rather than narrow. For example, a hospital whose average cost per discharge was $4,000 might get a 10 percent increase in a given year, increasing its maximum allowable payment under Medicare by $400 to $4,400. A hospital whose average cost per discharge was $2,000 would get an allowable payment of $2,200 in the following year, an increase of $200. Technically, the hospital with $4,000 costs per discharge might be subject to some penalty if its costs exceeded 112 percent of peer hospital costs per discharge, but this oversimplified example illustrates the basic inequity of the rate-of-increase limit.

Second, TEFRA used a methodology that did not fully reward efficiency. For example, if the allowable increase was 10 percent and the hospital held its rate of increase in costs to 5 percent, Medicare payments would increase by 7.5 percent. A similar hospital that claimed costs increased by 10 percent would receive the full 10 percent increase in Medicare allowable payment. Since the legitimacy of cost increases was not verified, TEFRA did not fully reward hospitals for holding down increases in costs over time through increased efficiency.

Congress recognized these limitations when TEFRA was being developed and viewed TEFRA as an intermediate step toward fundamental reform. Under the terms of the TEFRA legislation, the Secretary of Health and Human Services was directed to design a plan under which Medicare would pay hospitals prospectively and to submit this proposal by the end of 1982. It indicated that the new system should provide long-range payment reforms with built-in incentives for hospital efficiency.

Medicare Prospective Payment, 1983

In October 1982, as the TEFRA reimbursement provisions went into effect, Secretary of Health and Human Services Richard Schweiker announced the administration's intention to reform Medicare hospital payment policies by switching to prospective payment based on DRGs. Under the proposal, a national payment level would be determined for each of the 467 DRG categories, and every hospital would be paid the same rate for each diagnosis. Direct teaching costs and capital costs were to be "passed through" or paid based on cost, and adjustments in DRG rates were proposed to compensate for wage rate differences and indirect teaching costs (Schweiker 1982). Thus, as instructed in TEFRA, the administration delivered to Congress a prospective payment plan for Medicare.

PPS Goals

Secretary Schweiker's report to Congress included five major PPS goals. The first was to establish Medicare as a prudent buyer of services in the hospital market. Under cost-based reimbursement, Medicare paid hospitals whatever they legitimately claimed as costs for a particular service. In his report to Congress, for example, Schweiker stated that "an examination of Medicare records shows that payments for treating a heart attack average $1,500 at one hospital and $9,000 at another with no apparent difference in quality. Likewise Medicare payments for hip replacements can vary from $2,100 to $8,200 and payments for cataract removal vary from $450 to $2,800" (Schweiker 1982). TEFRA had done little to change the variability in payment rates across hospitals; therefore, PPS was designed to eliminate unjustifiable differences in medical practice and hospital pricing behavior by paying similar prices for comparable products.

A second goal of PPS was to reduce the rate of increase in federal Medicare expenditures. In his testimony before the Senate Finance Committee, Secretary Schweiker explained that "Medicare expenditures for hospital care have averaged a 19 percent increase each year between 1979 and 1982." He explained that even after general economic inflation slowed to 3.9 percent during 1982, overall hospital costs increased at a rate of over 12.6 percent. Controlling hospital costs quickly became a budgetary issue, since rising hospital costs constrain "the ability of the federal government to fund other health programs" (Schweiker 1983). A third goal was to ensure predictability in Medicare payments. Announcing payment rates in advance was intended to allow hospitals and Medicare to estimate their future budget requirements (Schweiker 1982). The fourth goal was to implement a payment system that would be less burdensome than cost-based reimbursement. Under cost-based reimbursement, hospitals were required to submit annual cost reports, which hospital administrators regarded as unnecessary regulation and an enormous burden. In addition, the reporting requirements under TEFRA were even greater than those under cost-based reimbursement. Under TEFRA, hospitals submitted the old cost reports with additional reports verifying that per-case limits had been recognized. PPS was expected to be relatively easy to administer and implement.

Finally, adoption of a prospective payment system was expected to encourage hospitals to operate more efficiently (Schweiker 1982). Under PPS, hospitals are paid a fixed amount for each case. They are permitted to keep any surplus resulting from cases in which the costs of treatment are less than the DRG payment, but they are forced to absorb a loss when the cost of a case exceeds the DRG payment. This system creates a powerful incentive to treat patients in the least costly manner possible. The financial rewards are greater under PPS than under TEFRA, and the penalties more onerous.

The Medicare PPS

The proposal was controversial. The health insurance industry expressed concern that the Medicare-only approach would result in costs being shifted to the privately insured. The AHA, which had proposed its own prospective plan, worried about specific provisions but generally supported a switch from the TEFRA system to prospective payment. Washington pundits predicted that since the TEFRA provisions already enacted accomplished the budget savings needed in fiscal year 1984 (the DRG proposal was designed to achieve no additional budget savings), Congress would do little more than discuss the prospective payment plan.

Three months after DHHS forwarded a prospective payment bill to Congress, the Medicare Prospective Payment System was signed into law. This swift action occurred for several reasons. Congressional staff remembered the delay that the Carter bill had encountered in moving through multiple committees and felt that only speedy action would prevent vested interests from getting organized and defeating the bill. Second, the legislation was attached to a piece of legislation that was required to pass. The Social Security program was in imminent danger of going bankrupt, and a consensus plan to ensure the fiscal solvency of this popular program was selected as the legislative vehicle for the Medicare hospital PPS. The final bill was approved on March 24, 1983. Nearly all of the public attention was focused on the provisions that would ensure the fiscal solvency of the Social Security program; virtually no media attention was given to the changes it represented for the hospital sector.

Congress made a number of modifications to the original proposal (Iglehart 1983b). As adopted by Congress in the spring of 1983 the Medicare Prospective Payment System had the following features:

- Hospitals were to be paid a prospectively determined payment rate for each hospital patient, with 467 different payment rates based on DRGs. A hospital's payment rate was not to be based on its own cost experience or on the scope of services provided.

- Payment rates were to increase each year at the rate of increase in the hospital market basket index plus one percentage point until 1986, at which time increases in the payment rates were left to the discretion of the Secretary of Health and Human Services.

- Payment rates were to be adjusted for differences in wage levels in the surrounding community and for geographic location.

- Cases involving an unusually long length of stay or abnormally high costs, called "outlier cases," were reimbursed separately. Fewer than 6 percent of all cases could be defined as outliers.

- Certain hospitals and services were excluded from PPS, including hospital outpatient services, as well as certain rehabilitative, psychiatric, and long-term care services in distinct parts of community hospitals. Children's hospitals, rehabilitation hospitals, psychiatric hospitals, and long-term care hospitals were also exempt.

- Direct medical education expenses were to be reimbursed at cost. Indirect expenses of medical education were to be paid on the basis of a formula. The formula increased hospitals payments by 11.57 percent for each full-time equivalent intern and resident per ten beds.

- Capital costs, including interest expenses, depreciation, and rent, were to be reimbursed at cost.

- The DRG rates were to be recalibrated every four years beginning in 1986 to account for changes in costs per discharge that were attributable to changes in medical practice patterns and availability of new technologies.

- Each state was required to establish a medical peer review group, called the professional review organization (PRO), to oversee quality and monitor lengths of stay.

- PPS began on 1 October 1983. Hospitals started under the system with the beginning of their accounting year.

- PPS was to be phased in over a four-year period to allow hospitals to adjust to the new system. During this period the hospital received a payment rate that was to be a blend of the DRG payment rate and a payment rate based on the hospital's own costs (called the hospital specific cost per case).

- The PPS legislation established a Prospective Payment Assessment Commission (ProPAC) to oversee PPS and to make recommendations to modify the system. The legislation also mandated a number of studies and reports to be conducted by DHHS.

- States with their own system of regulating hospital rates for patients were exempted subject to meeting conditions on performance, such as saving the Medicare program at least as much as PPS. Approved state programs had to cover 75 percent of inpatient revenues and ensure that access to hospital services was not impaired.

Many of these provisions were altered in subsequent years as the result of new analysis or political or economic pressures.

Measurement of the Hospital Patient Case Mix

A critical issue in PPS concerns the case mix measurement system. DHHS considered several such measures before making a recommendation to Congress, including DRGs (Fetter et al. 1977), severity of illness (Horn 1981), patient management paths (Young 1979; Young, Swinkola, and Zorn 1982), and disease staging (Gonnella and Goran 1975).

In order to evaluate alternative patient classification systems, the department established four criteria. First, it sought to use a system that would apply to all patients. Some of the alternative case mix measures could not classify all patients; if these alternative case mix measures had been selected, the department would have had to develop an alternative payment system for the cases not covered by the case mix system. Second, the department was looking for a case mix adjustment system that classified patients based on explicit guidelines, requiring minimal discretionary judgment. The greater the judgment required, the greater the possibility that the system would be "gamed" in order to maximize payment (Simborg 1981). Third, the system had to be implemented at low cost. Because Medicare pays for approximately 10 million discharges per year, case mix systems that require major changes in the administration of the program would increase costs substantially. Fourth, the department sought a system that already had been used to classify hospital inpatients for payment purposes.

The department chose to use the DRG case mix measurement system, the only system to fit all four criteria. DRGs had been used both to set per-case limits under TEFRA and to classify New Jersey hospital patients under a Medicare waiver since 1980 (Iglehart 1982b; Merrill 1984; Vladeck 1984). The use of DRGs was appealing because rates could be based upon information already collected by the government; moreover, minimum judgment was required in classifying patients into DRGs.

Calculating the Payment Rates

Under a fully phased-in PPS the amount a hospital receives for a discharge is the product of two numbers: the DRG relative weight and a national average cost per discharge, called the standardized base payment. The standardized base payment includes adjustments to account for the hospital's rural or urban location and local wage rates (Vladeck 1984) and other factors which Congress can determine. The calculations performed, data used to derive these values, and the method of determining a payment amount for each individual DRG are discussed in greater detail below.

The weights of the DRGs reflect the resource intensity of each DRG.

Weights are the same for every hospital. They were originally calculated using the Medicare Provider Analysis and Review (MedPAR) file, which includes charge data on a sample of Medicare patients, and the Medicare Cost Reports (MCRs). The MedPAR file contains clinical and charge information on a 20 percent sample of all Medicare hospital claims. MCRs contain hospital-specific cost information submitted to Medicare by all hospitals. Non-Medicare discharge records for Maryland and Michigan hospitals were also used to derive weights for those DRGs for which Medicare patient files did not contain enough patients in a specific DRG. These are primarily maternity and pediatric cases, which rarely involve the aged majority of Medicare patients. After combining these two data sources, the Health Care Financing Association (HCFA) calculated an overall average cost per case and a DRG-specific average cost. The DRG-specific average cost was then divided by the overall average cost per case to determine the relative weight of each DRG (Vladeck 1984).

In 1986, DRG weights were recalibrated by HCFA using charge data from the 1984 Patent Bill (PATBILL) file. This data file contained a 100 percent sample of Medicare hospital discharges. HCFA contended that these data were more complete and would reduce the number of low-volume DRGs and allow construction of 1986 DRG weights that more accurately reflected relative resource use. Thus the weights reflect the charge for delivering care for a particular DRG as compared with the overall average charge for all Medicare cases. Table 3.2 provides a sample of DRGs and their relative weights.

The weight is multiplied by an adjusted standardized base payment. The standardized amount is essentially the average Medicare per-case cost in 1981 adjusted for inflation. Further adjustments to the standardized payment amount are made to determine a rate for a specific hospital. One adjustment is for the effect of location. DHHS is required to develop a separate standardized payment amount for urban and rural hospitals. In 1984, hospitals located in urban areas were paid rates approximately 20 percent higher than those paid to hospitals located in rural areas. The other adjustment to the base payment concerns the prevailing wage for hospital workers in the geographic area in which the hospital is located. Since approximately 70 percent of a hospital's costs are attributable to labor costs (Freeland, Anderson, and Schendler 1979), and other costs vary with the cost of labor, variations in the cost of this input affect the cost of a discharge significantly (see table 3.3).

The process of adjusting the payment for a particular DRG for differences in wage levels is as follows:

1. $\begin{array}{c} \text{79.15\% of urban} \\ \text{or rural payment} \\ \text{amount} \end{array}$ $\times$ $\begin{array}{c} \text{Area} \\ \text{wage} \\ \text{index} \end{array}$ $+$ $\begin{array}{c} \text{10.85\% of urban or} \\ \text{rural standardized} \\ \text{amount} \end{array}$ $=$ $\begin{array}{c} \text{ADJUSTED} \\ \text{AMOUNT} \end{array}$

   $\underbrace{\hspace{5cm}}_{\text{LABOR-RELATED PORTION}}$ $\underbrace{\hspace{5cm}}_{\begin{array}{c}\text{NONLABOR-RELATED}\\\text{PORTION}\end{array}}$

2. $\begin{array}{c} \text{ADJUSTED} \\ \text{AMOUNT} \end{array}$ $\times$ $\begin{array}{c} \text{DRG} \\ \text{WEIGHT} \end{array}$ $=$ $\begin{array}{c} \text{DRG} \\ \text{PAYMENT} \end{array}$

To calculate a payment level, the payment amount is divided into a labor-related and a nonlabor-related portion. The labor-related portion of the payment amount is multiplied by the area wage index of the geographic area in which the hospital is located. This product is added to the nonlabor component of the payment amount. The sum is an adjusted payment amount that reflects differences in production costs attributable to differences in wages. Adjusted rates are updated and published annually by the Secretary of Health and Human Services.

The adjusted base payment amount is then multiplied by the DRG relative weight to determine the hospital's payment level for a particular DRG. Table 3.4 shows the derivation of a payment amount in 1984 for DRG 236, fracture of the hip and pelvis, for hospitals located in Boston; Charleston, South Carolina; and rural Kentucky. As the table shows, payment levels for a particular DRG can vary by several thousand dollars depending on geographic location and wage rates.

Increases in Payment Rates over Time

One of the most important features of PPS was a provision establishing changes in the DRG payment rates over time. This provision affects the long-term savings of the system and represented the federal government's determination to control outlays for hospital services under the Medicare program.

According to the original legislation, for the three years following the legislation's adoption payment rates were to increase by the market basket inflation rate plus 1 percent for new technology and services (the so-called intensity factor). This adjustment was intended to reimburse hospitals for increases in the cost of inputs purchased by hospitals and to allow an additional 1 percent for technological changes and improvements in quality. Beginning in fiscal year 1986, the legislation authorized the Secretary of Health and Human Services to set the rate of increase, taking into consideration the recommendations of ProPAC.

In practice, this feature was of such keen political interest that it has since been determined annually through congressional amendments to the original legislation. Table 3.5 displays the update factor recommended by the administration and by ProPAC for fiscal year 1986 in contrast with

Table 3.3. Community Hospital Relative Weights by Expense Category, 1977

Expense Category	Relative Weight
Payroll expenses and employee benefits	
Payroll expenses (wages and salaries)	51.69
Employee benefits	7.22
	58.01
Professional fees	
Medical	4.46
Other (legal, auditing, consulting, etc.)	0.52
	4.98
Capital	
Depreciation	4.01
Building and fixed equipment	2.58
Movable equipment	1.43
Interest	2.01
Working capital	0.41
Capital debt	1.60
	6.02
Hospital malpractice insurance premiums	2.00
Food	
Purchases at early stages of distribution	1.57
Purchases at later stages of distribution	1.56
	3.13
Fuel and other utilities	
Fuel oil and coal	0.94
Electricity	0.67
Natural gas	0.50
Water and sanitary services	0.31
	2.42
Other	
Drugs	2.48
Chemicals and cleaning products	1.88
Surgical and medical instruments and appliances	1.78
Rubber and miscellaneous plastics	1.62
Business travel and motor freight	1.51
Apparel and textiles	1.45
Business services	4.12
All other miscellaneous expenses	7.70
	22.54
Total	100.00

Source: Freeland, Anderson, and Schendler 1979.

Table 3.4. An Example of Derivation of DRG Payment for DRG 236, Hip and Pelvis Fracture, Fiscal Year 1984

	$\left(\begin{array}{c}\text{Labor} \\ \text{Portion}\end{array} \times \begin{array}{c}\text{Wage} \\ \text{Index}\end{array}\right)$		$+ \left(\begin{array}{c}\text{Nonlabor} \\ \text{Portion}\end{array}\right) =$	$\left(\begin{array}{c}\text{Adjusted} \\ \text{Standardized} \\ \text{Amount}\end{array} \times \begin{array}{c}\text{Adjusted} \\ \text{DRG} \\ \text{Weight}\end{array}\right) =$		$\begin{array}{c}\text{DRG} \\ \text{Payment}\end{array}$
Boston	$2,770.25	1.0949	$729.75	$3,762.89	1.3855	$5,218.49
Charleston, S.C.	$2,770.25	1.0262	$729.75	$3,572.58	1.3855	$4,949.81
Kentucky, rural areas	$2,216.20	0.8154	$583.80	$2,390.88	1.3855	$3,312.57

Note: These estimates were derived using 1984 standardized payments, wage indexes, and DRG weights. The labor portion is derived by multiplying the national standardized amount ($3,500 for urban areas, $2,800 for rural areas) by the percentage of costs represented by labor (79.15%). The nonlabor portion is derived by multiplying the national (urban or rural) standardized amount by the percentage of costs represented by nonlabor functions (20.85%).
Source: Senate Committee on Finance 1983.

Table 3.5. PPS Increases, 1984–1989

Year	Market Basket plus 1%	ProPAC Recommendation	Actual[a]
1984	5.9	—	—
1985	5.0	—	3.4
1986	4.1	1.5	0.3[b]
1987	4.5	1.9	1.1
1988	5.7	2.3	0.9[b]
1989	6.4	4.2	3.3[c]

Sources: HCFA, personal communication to G. Anderson, 1988; ProPAC 1988.
[a]Overall increase approved by Congress.
[b]Adjusted for the number of months the PPS update factor was in effect during a PPS year.
[c]Based on current law estimate of "Market basket—2.1."

the final legislative determination by Congress, later signed into law by the president. The annual rate of increase in the payment rates has become a political football, with the final decision based largely on federal budgetary considerations.

Outlier Policy

Although policy officials designing PPS believed that DRGs were the best available case mix measure, they were concerned that using DRGs would result in substantial underpayment for certain patients. One concern was that because DRG payments are based on averages, DRG-based reimbursement would fail to pay adequately for exceptionally high-cost patients (Eisenberg 1984; Omenn and Conrad 1984). A small hospital that admitted an unusually costly patient could conceivably go broke if it received only the DRG rate for that case. In addition, without an adjustment for very expensive services, a hospital would have little incentive to admit and treat patients requiring an array of intensive and costly services.

For these reasons, a separate system for reimbursing hospitals for patients with a long length of stay and/or high costs was established. A hospital receives the flat DRG payment for patients whose length of stay is within the limited number of days set for each DRG by DHHS (Vladeck 1984). These limits, which are based on the geometric mean lengths of stay, are illustrated for the first thirty-five DRGs in table 3.2. Once a patient's length of stay exceeds a minimum number of days, the hospital will receive a payment for each additional day the patient is in the hospital.

An adjustment is also made for cost outliers. These are cases in which costs for that particular case are above some threshold amount. An additional payment equal to the marginal cost of care beyond the outlier criteria is provided to the hospital.

Teaching Costs

After a hospital's aggregate payment for all DRGs is determined, an additional allowance is added for both direct and indirect teaching costs. Direct teaching costs (residents' salaries, nursing, costs of administering the residency program, costs associated with operating other health profession training programs) are paid using cost-based reimbursement, a payment totally separate from the DRG payment amount. Under cost-based reimbursement and TEFRA, hospitals received reimbursement for the direct costs of medical education attributable to the hospital's share of Medicare patients. This was continued under PPS.

During the debate over implementation of PPS there was concern about the ability of the DRG case mix system to account fully for factors contributing to costs unique to teaching hospitals. Teaching hospitals, particularly major teaching hospitals, tend to be significantly more expensive than their nonteaching counterparts. Patients requiring the specialized and costly services of teaching hospitals may be more severely ill than others. In addition, teaching hospitals produce multiple products, including training of physicians, nurses, and allied health professionals and unsponsored research, for which they are not paid explicitly. Also, many teaching hospitals treat a disproportionate share of indigent patients. To account for these incremental costs, policy officials made an additional allowance over and above the DRG payment rate. This allowance had roots in the treatment of teaching costs under Section 223. Under Section 223 the cost ceiling was increased by 5.79 percent for each 0.1 full-time equivalent interns and residents per hospital bed. PPS doubled this allowance and increased hospital DRG payments by 11.59 percent for each intern and resident per ten beds. Subsequent legislation has reduced this amount. The indirect medical education allowance is calculated by dividing the ratio of interns and residents per bed by 0.1. The result is then multiplied by an adjustment factor. This product is then multiplied by the sum of all the DRG payments to yield an indirect teaching cost payment.

$$1. \ \frac{\text{NUMBER OF INTERNS} + \text{RESIDENTS/NUMBER OF BEDS}}{0.1} \times 0.1159$$

$$= \text{TEACHING ADJUSTMENT}$$

2. TEACHING   ×   HOSPITAL'S AGGREGATE   =   INDIRECT TEACHING
   ADJUSTMENT   DRG PAYMENT AMOUNT   COST PAYMENT

Capital Costs

The 1983 PPS legislation also continued the cost-based reimbursement of capital expenses such as interest expenses, taxes, insurance, depreciation, and rent. This was intended to be a temporary measure until a new PPS could be developed for capital. Since 1983, various pieces of legislation have addressed the issue of capital costs. Hospitals are no longer able to "pass through" capital costs at a 100 percent rate. Legislated charges have instituted a copayment system according to which Medicare pays increasingly less and hospitals are responsible for increasingly more. For example, under legislation passed in 1987 the Medicare program pays only 85 percent of capital costs in 1989. The incorporation of capital costs into PPS has been repeatedly prohibited.

Recalibration

In order to account for changes in patterns of medical practice, any payment system must be flexible enough to be adjusted intermittently. This is true because medical practice and technology are constantly evolving. Payments may change when new technologies prove to be more or less costly than the current approach. For example, the development of lithotripters may change the cost of treating patients with kidney stones. In addition, standard treatment regimens may be altered by the medical community, resulting in either an increase or a decrease in the cost of treating cases. For example, the standard length of stay of myocardial infarction patients has dropped considerably because of new consensus in the medical community that patients with heart attacks should be discharged earlier. The legislation included a provision calling for recalibration of DRG weights at least every four years to take into account changes in medicine, medical practice patterns, and technology. Subsequent legislation required that recalibration be done on an annual basis.

The PPS legislation called for the establishment of an independent body of commissioners to oversee the implementation of the payment system, to monitor its progress, and to make recommendations on re-calibration needs. This group, ProPAC, also advises the department on technical matters and coverage issues related to PPS.

PROs

When the department proposed that Medicare adopt a DRG-based PPS, it recognized that PPS offered incentives that would influence patterns of medical practice and the delivery of care significantly. Some anticipated that the new payment system would adversely affect the quality of care delivered. For example, PPS created incentives to unbundle hospital ser-vices (Stern and Epstein 1985). In order to decrease the costs of treating a case, some physicians would choose to perform diagnostic tests or other procedures outside the hospital setting, either prior to admission or fol-lowing discharge.

Other anticipated results of PPS included a decrease in lengths of stay and an increase in admissions (Davis et al. 1985; Stern and Epstein 1985). Some were concerned that hospitals would discharge patients prema-turely, given the economic incentive to keep costs below the Medicare payment rate. While shortened lengths of stay are not necessarily harm-ful, in some cases quality of care could be jeopardized. Similarly, there was some concern that to increase payment, patients requiring extensive treatment for multiple conditions would be admitted and treated for one diagnosis, discharged, and readmitted in a second DRG. This would lead not only to double payments for the same patient but also to a decline in the quality of patient care (Anderson and Steinberg 1984b).

To monitor these changes, the legislation established a system of peer review organizations. The PROs replaced the previously established Professional Standards Review Organizations. Like the PSROs, they are responsible for monitoring the quality of care. Their charge is to review the validity of diagnoses; the appropriateness of admissions, discharges, and transfers; and the nature and management of outlier cases (Congress 1983).

Phase-in

The legislation establishing PPS did not mandate immediate application of these rates. Instead, a four-year transition period was established to ease the impact of these changes. This period was later extended, and the transition was complete by November 1987. During the transition period a declining proportion of Medicare payments would be based on the hospitals' own costs, and an increasing percentage would be based on DRG rates. The transition was necessary for two reasons. First, this approach enabled hospitals to adjust to the new payment method by adjusting their management practices. Second, the transition period would allow the federal government to monitor cost and management changes and to refine the system as needed before full implementation.

State Waivers

Several states (including Maryland, Massachusetts, New Jersey, and New York) developed state hospital cost containment programs, with commissions authorized to approve hospital rates and/or budgets. Under the 1972 amendments to Medicare, federal funds were used to develop these alternatives to cost-based payment systems. Waivers from Medicare permitted payment of hospitals on state-determined payment principles rather than cost-based principles.

With passage of PPS, states were permitted to continue operating under a Medicare waiver provided that:

- the state's system applied to all nonfederal acute-care hospitals;
- the state's system applied to at least 75 percent of all inpatient revenues (or expenses) for the state;
- the state provided assurance that payers, hospital employees, and patients would be treated equitably;
- the state provided assurance that its system would not result in greater Medicare expenditures over a thirty-six month period;
- the state did not preclude HMOs or competitive medical plans from negotiating directly with hospitals concerning payment for inpatient services;
- the system was operated by the state or an entity designated by state law;
- the system used a prospective payment methodology;
- the system provided hospital cost reports to the federal DHHS;
- the state provided assurance that the system would not result in admission practices that would reduce treatment to uninsured, low-income, high-cost, or emergency patients;
- the state did not reduce payments without sixty days notice to HCFA and hospitals; and
- the state provided assurance that it had consulted with local officials concerning the system's effect on public hospitals.

An Initial Evaluation of the Medicare PPS

Experience with the Medicare PPS has been sufficiently short that it is difficult to draw definitive conclusions about its long-term impact. It is a dramatic departure from years of cost-based reimbursement that provided no incentive for hospitals to economize or improve productivity. Clearly, it has caught the attention of hospital management and physicians—not only in the United States but in many other industrialized nations.

One major lesson of the U.S. experience is the susceptibility of any system to political and social forces. The driving desire to obtain federal budgetary savings has quickly transformed PPS from a "revenue-neutral" device aimed at improving fairness and rewarding efficiency to a cost containment device.

Even though the evidence is quite preliminary, it would appear that this new set of economic incentives has had a major impact on the hospital sector. Hospital management is quite sensitive to the cost implications of decisions regarding acquisition of new equipment or development of a new service. The medical community is quite familiar with PPS and in fact tends to overattribute all changes in the health care system to DRGs. It has changed the attitude that physicians can make decisions about patient care without regard to the financial consequences and has inculcated an attitude that someone is looking over the shoulder of the hospital wanting justification for keeping the patient in the hospital another day or ordering an expensive test.

It has mobilized changes on the part of other payers. As chapter 4 discusses, many state Medicaid programs have adopted PPS for Medicaid patients. Chapter 8 also notes the marketing of PPOs to major employers, at least in part to avoid any cost shifting onto privately insured patients.

What is perhaps most significant, in a short period of time PPS has established itself as an entrenched part of the health financing system. Predictions that it would collapse of its own weight from excess complexity have not been borne out. It has been accepted by patients, providers, and payers—with varying degrees of concern. It appears well on its way to having many long-term effects on the health care delivery system in the United States.

The primary objective of PPS was to reduce the rate of increase in federal budgetary expenditures for services provided to elderly and disabled Medicare beneficiaries. It was also hoped that Medicare hospital payment reform would result in slower inflation in hospital costs for all patients. Since Medicare payments to hospitals represent only 35 percent of total hospital payments, however, it is not clear how changes in payment rates for Medicare patients only will affect overall hospital cost performance.

At the time of passage, many analysts predicted that the new system would lead to substantial changes in hospital behavior and performance (Davis, Anderson, and Steinberg 1984; Lave 1984; Vladeck 1984). Anticipated effects included the following:

- Shorter hospital stays (Davis, Anderson, and Steinberg 1984)
- Increased readmissions of Medicare beneficiaries (Anderson and Steinberg 1984a)
- Shifting of costs to privately insured patients (Meyer and Johnson 1983)
- Elimination of nonpaying or nonprofitable services, such as patient education services (Lave 1984)
- Shifting some care, such as preadmission diagnostic testing, to an outpatient basis (Lave 1984)
- Dumping or transferring to other institutions patients with higher than average severity of illness within a given DRG (Horn et al. 1985)
- DRG creep, or an increasing tendency of hospitals to classify patients in DRG categories with higher payment rates (Lave 1984; Simborg 1981)
- Increased reluctance or refusal to care for uninsured patients because of reduced ability to cross-subsidize such care from other patient revenues (Davis et al. 1984)
- Diminished quality of care as hospitals cut corners or physicians were pressured to forgo expensive diagnostic testing or treatment regimens (Davis et al. 1984)
- Reduced acquisition, diffusion, and utilization of cost-increasing technology (Anderson and Steinberg 1984b)
- Increased diversification of hospital operations, including moving into long-term care services such as home health services or nursing homes to provide care in other settings following earlier hospital discharges (Lave 1984)
- Increased interaction between hospital administrators and organized medical staffs, including acceleration of trends toward salaried service chiefs in community hospitals and greater external scrutiny of physicians' activities (Vladeck, 1984)

Early experience with the Medicare PPS confirms only some of these concerns. Chapter 8 reviews the evidence to date of the impact of the Medicare PPS and other cost containment measures in slowing the rate of increase in hospital costs nationwide.

Many of the predictions appear to have been borne out. Hospital lengths of stay of the elderly have shortened dramatically (Davis et al. 1985; HCFA 1986b), and hospitals do seem to have upgraded the classification of patient diagnosis, leading to higher DRG payment (HCFA

1986b). It should be noted that several concerns have not been supported by the initial response of the hospital sector. Hospital admissions of the elderly have not increased but rather have gone down slightly (Davis et al. 1985). Financial failure of hospitals has not occurred on a widespread basis; instead profit margins have gone up initially (Iglehart 1986). There does not appear to be massive cost shifting to the private sector. However, it is possible that these concerns will be substantiated in subsequent years.

The major issue at dispute is whether PPS is having an adverse effect on the quality of care. Some investigations have found that Medicare patients are being discharged "quicker and sicker" (GAO 1985a). While in and of itself this phenomenon may not be undesirable, many communities do not offer appropriate postdischarge services, such as home care for frail patients. Even when such services are available, many Medicare enrollees do not have sufficient resources to purchase them.

Major Lessons

The evolution of hospital cost initiatives at the federal level demonstrates the importance of political forces and the environment in shaping legislative action. In the mid and late seventies the political will to constrain hospital costs did not exist. Repeatedly the executive branch and its analysts documented that hospital inflation was out of hand and offered proposals to curb costs. Congress, however, elected not to regulate and chose to give the hospitals another chance to restrain costs voluntarily.

The political resistance to regulation at the federal level can be explained by several factors. First, consumer concern over rising health costs was not significant enough to generate political pressure from constituents. Second, the hospital industry was aggressive and vocal in its opposition. Third, regulation of an industry whose quality of care affected life and death was an uncomfortable extension of federal authority for many members of Congress.

What then changed the course of Congress's policy with regard to hospitals? The election of Reagan as president and the tremendous pressures generated by his administration and newly elected members of Congress to cut the federal budget changed the political environment. Looming federal deficits caused by tax cuts and substantial increases in military spending left the domestic budget to take the brunt of reductions in federal spending. Because of the strength of the senior citizens' lobby and their voting clout, the largest domestic expenditure, Social Security, remained untouchable; Medicare became an obvious target for savings.

Several factors appear to have come together to create a political climate conducive to enactment of the first TEFRA limits, followed by the DRG payment system. First, totally independent of health policy, the reconciliation process put budget cuts on a rapid legislative cycle and reduced the deliberation process. The Reagan administration used this legislative vehicle to enact savings in the total budget in 1981 and 1982. Second, when Congress was required by the reconciliation process to make deep cuts in domestic program spending, Medicare was so large it could not be avoided. This was especially true in 1982, when TEFRA was enacted, since large savings in the non-Medicare domestic programs had already been achieved in the Omnibus Reconciliation Act of 1981. Third, if Medicare was to be cut, hospital payment reductions were politically more acceptable than benefit reductions that directly affected the elderly. Politically, it could be argued that the cuts were only trimming excessive "fat" in hospitals and would not harm the elderly. And finally, by 1982 Congress was tired of the hospital industry's promises to restrain costs voluntarily.

The successful enactment of TEFRA and PPS represents more, however, than just successful political timing. The second key to the success of these initiatives was that they focused on payments for Medicare only and did not attempt to institute all-payer controls. It appears that Congress was more willing to act as a "prudent Medicare purchaser" than as a public regulator of the hospital industry. TEFRA and the DRG system of PPS both limit payment for care for Medicare beneficiaries, as did earlier Section 223 limits. But since all of these limits did not apply to all payers, responsibility for the fiscal health of the hospital industry has not been added to the public agenda. It is politically acceptable to control Medicare costs in order to contain the federal budget. It is not politically acceptable to regulate the hospital industry to control overall hospital cost inflation. Federal initiatives directed at the latter goal will require a major change in the current political climate.

Future Directions

In the years since the passage of the PPS legislation there has been considerable discussion about specific provisions and the subsequent implementation of PPS. Each year since it was adopted, Congress has discussed various provisions of PPS and made modifications to it; however, the system still poses many problems for policymakers, administrators, physicians, and patients.

The Aggregate Rate of Increase in DRG Payments

One of the stated goals of PPS was to establish in advance how much hospitals would be paid for each admission. Based on this goal, Congress developed a formula approach in the original legislation to adjust payments in subsequent years. When the prospective payment legislation was originally passed, PPS payment rates were permitted to increase for the first three years at a rate equivalent to the hospital market basket inflation rate plus 1 percent for new technology and services.

After the first year the actual allowable rate of increase has been lower because of administration recommendations and congressional action. Each year the president's budget has requested an increase in hospital payment levels that has amounted to much less than the market basket inflation rate plus 1 percent. ProPAC has proposed rates of increase based upon objective factors similar to the market basket plus 1 percent. These recommended rates have been substantially higher than those proposed by the president.

After considerable debate between Congress and the administration, Congress agreed to payment rate increases somewhat greater than those proposed by the administration but less than the automatic increases established by the PPS legislation and those proposed by ProPAC. An important consideration in their deliberations was the profit margins enjoyed by hospitals during the early years of PPS. By adjusting Medicare payment rates for budgetary reasons and to lower hospital profit margins, the administration and Congress abandoned the original goal of establishing predictability in hospital revenues.

Hospitals would be able to plan better if the system were less subject to annual political negotiations. One approach would be to return to an objective method for establishing the appropriate rate of increase. This method could be adopted once the hospital profit margins return to long-run averages. The objective method should consider inflation, productivity gains, technological development, and other factors. The methodology developed by ProPAC to establish the rate of increase is a good beginning; it takes into account not only changes in input costs but also changes in productivity, scientific and technological advancement, changes in case mix and severity within DRGs, and site substitution. Table 3.6 presents the methodology used by ProPAC to determine the appropriate rate of increase for 1990. This computation is highly technical and not based on policy or budgetary judgments.

If it is impossible to avoid political negotiations over the rate of increase in DRG payment rates, rates should at a minimum be determined in advance over a longer period of time—say, three years. This would provide hospitals with a greater ability to plan for future years and would remove the current year-to-year negotiations.

Patient Care

The debate concerning the long-term viability of PPS has centered on its ability to set fair prices for specific patient care services. There is concern that the payment system both recognize the variability in costs associated

Table 3.6. **Estimated PPS Update Factors for Fiscal Year 1990 under ProPAC Recommendations**

Total Update Factor	
Average update factor	4.9%
Large urban	5.0
Other urban	4.5
Rural	5.6
Components of the Update Factor	
Components applied to all hospitals	
Fiscal year 1990 market basket forecast[a]	5.7%
Correction for fiscal year 1989 forecast error[b]	0.6
Components of discretionary adjustment factor	
Scientific and technological advancement[c]	—
Productivity[c]	—
Total discretionary adjustment factor	0.0
Case mix change	
Total DRG case mix index change	−3.0
Real DRG case mix index change	1.5
Within-DRG patient complexity	0.8
Net adjustment for case mix change	−0.7
Components applied to urban hospitals only	
Third-year phased reduction to standardized amounts	
Adjustment for large urban areas	−0.8
Adjustment for other urban areas	−0.8
Urban population differential	
Adjustment for large urban areas	0.2
Adjustment for other urban areas	−0.3

Source: ProPAC 1989.

[a]Forecast of ProPAC-recommended PPS market basket by Data Resources, Inc.

[b]The market basket forecast used for the fiscal year 1989 update was 5.4 percent. The most recent fiscal year 1989 forecast is 6.1 percent. The full difference is not adjusted because no correction is made for errors in forecasting hospital industry wages.

[c]In ProPAC's judgment, the added costs for scientific and technological advancement should be funded by increases in hospital productivity; therefore, these components of the update factor sum to zero.

with treating patients with different medical conditions and appropriately adjust for input cost differences across hospitals. Most of the discussion concerning case mix has focused on the ability of the DRG system to measure the resources required to treat a particular patient. The system has been criticized for incorrectly grouping dissimilar patients into the same DRG (Horn et al. 1986a), for not being sufficiently robust to adjust to changing medical practices (Anderson and Steinberg 1984b), for being susceptible to DRG upcoding (Simborg 1981), and for inappropriately rewarding or penalizing hospitals for the use of certain procedures (Anderson and Steinberg 1986; Omenn and Conrad 1984). Some claim that DRGs do not adequately define or measure the products of teaching and tertiary care hospitals, which may have a more complicated case mix than other hospitals (Horn et al. 1985). The most frequently mentioned modification is a means of incorporating a measure of differences in the complexity of illness. Related case mix issues include outlier policy and recalibration.

Alternative Case Mix Measures

Since the inception of Medicare's PPS, policymakers, researchers, hospital administrators, and others have questioned the ability of the DRG system to measure a hospital's case mix adequately. Researchers have developed several other case mix measures in an attempt to introduce a more medically meaningful case mix measure than DRGs into the Medicare program.

Alternative measures that have been proposed include severity of illness, patient management paths, and disease staging (Hornbrook 1982). The patient management categories and disease staging classification schemes are alike in several ways: both use physician panels, objective classification material, and readily available material. Neither include actual utilization of services as a basis for classification. The patient management categories were developed by Young to define and group homogeneous hospital patients (Young, Swinkola, and Zorn 1982). They link diagnostic groups and physician treatment decisions to estimate the relative cost of each patient category. Disease staging, developed by Gonnella, measures the severity of the patient's condition at a given point in time by defining five clinically identifiable stages in the progression of the disease (Gonnella and Goran 1975). Substages within each primary disease are also defined. One purpose of disease staging is to avoid confounding the patient's condition with the therapeutic response.

The most frequently suggested refinement to the DRG system is to incorporate a severity-of-illness (SOI) measure into PPS (Horn 1981). The original SOI measure assigned one of four severity scores to each patient upon or following discharge. The level of severity was determined by evaluating the patient's medical record along seven dimensions. A new computerized version of SOI uses objective criteria to assign patients a severity score.

Two studies comparing DRGs and alternative case mix measures found that the overall level of explanation is higher when the DRGs are combined with an alternative case mix measure. Both studies found that severity of illness in combination with DRGs explains more of the total variance in patient costs than DRGs alone or DRGs combined with disease staging (Berman 1986; Arthur Young 1986). However, until additional comparative studies are completed, it will be impossible to state conclusively which alternative case mix measure best explains the variance in hospital expenditures. It may be necessary to test the alternative case mix measures in real world situations.

Outlier Policy

PPS partially adjusts for an inadequate case mix classification system by providing an outlier payment. Patients whose length of stay or total covered charges adjusted to costs differ substantially from the mean length of stay or total cost for patients in their DRG are classified as outliers, and hospitals receive compensation for these unusual cases in addition to the DRG payment. A day outlier is defined as a patient whose length of stay exceeds the mean for the DRG by the lesser of a fixed number of days (eighteen in 1988) or a fixed number of standard deviations. A cost outlier is a patient whose total covered charges exceed the greater of a fixed dollar amount ($14,000 in 1988) or a fixed multiple of the PPS rate.

Under current policy, hospitals are losing an average of $7,000 per outlier case. This degree of financial loss increases the probability that particular patients will experience discrimination. The Rand Corporation developed the concept of "stop loss outliers." According to Rand's definition, an "optimal" outlier policy has the following characteristics:

- Hospitals could lose a certain amount on outliers; in insurance terms this is called a deductible.
- It would pay the hospital's full marginal costs (losses) in excess of a deductible amount.
- The dollar amount of the deductible would be the same for all cases.
- The dollar amount of the deductible would be set so that the sum of the marginal costs for all cases with losses above the deductible would completely exhaust the available budget for outlier payments.

This type of approach could protect both the hospitals and the patient.

Medicare does not adjust for short-length-of-stay outliers. The legislation did not mandate a short-length-of-stay outlier under PPS because it was believed that hospitals would admit a balance of both high- and low-cost patients within a DRG. This policy of admitting a mix of high- and low-cost patients would result in hospitals' making a profit on some patients and losing money on others. Thus, patients who remained in the hospital a short period of time would subsidize patients who remained a long time. As the program has evolved, however, this cross-subsidization has not occurred; instead, many hospital managers have responded to the incentives created by PPS by encouraging physicians to discharge patients according to the mean length of stay for their DRG. The decline in average length of stay among Medicare patients may be partially attributable to the fact that few patients stay in the hospital longer than the predicted average length of stay for their DRG.

To discourage inappropriately short lengths of stay, policymakers should consider establishing a short-length-of-stay outlier in which hospitals would not receive the entire DRG payment for patients whose stay is unusually short. A short-outlier policy would allow the Medicare program to recover some of the savings generated by short lengths of stay. In addition, hospitals would be discouraged from admitting a patient for a short period of time in order to receive the full DRG payment, thus reducing both the number of inappropriate admissions and the number of readmissions. New Jersey employs a version of the short-length-of-stay outlier.

Inner City Location

Most empirical studies of hospital costs have found that costs are higher in urban areas than in rural areas (Pettingill and Vertrees 1982). It is not surprising, therefore, that PPS payment rates are higher for hospitals located in urban areas than for rural hospitals. Recent studies have demonstrated that within an urban area, costs for an inner city hospital are higher than those for a suburban hospital (Anderson and Lave 1986; Ashby 1984). It may be necessary to subdivide urban areas into central city and suburban ring, creating three payment categories—urban, suburban, rural—based on location. This adjustment would reduce the adverse impact of PPS on hospitals located in the central city.

The Nonlabor Share

In most hospitals, wages and fringe benefits represent approximately two-thirds of the hospital's total budget (Freeland, Anderson, and Schendler 1979). The remaining one-third of the budget is used for drugs and equipment, food, utilities, and other services necessary for the provision of hospital care. For these expenditures there is no adjustment for regional variations in costs. The wage index can be used as a proxy to adjust for some of these goods and services but not others (HCFA 1986b). More research is warranted to determine whether there is significant variation in the cost of these nonlabor inputs and to develop adjustments for any variation in the nonlabor portion of hospital expenditures.

Summary

An improved PPS would do the following:

- Incorporate a complexity of illness measure in addition to DRGs
- Adjust for both long- and short-length-of stay outliers
- Incorporate adjustments for nonlabor costs and inner city locations

Financing Other Products

Many hospitals are multiproduct firms providing biomedical research, technological development, care for the poor, training for health care professionals, and other products in addition to patient care. Traditionally hospitals have subsidized many of these products by using patient care dollars provided by third-party payers, including Medicare. PPS substantially reduces the ability of hospitals to subsidize these products using patient care revenues. Other hospital payment reforms also reduce the ability of hospitals to cross-subsidize these products and services. Thus policymakers are required to investigate alternative sources of financing for these services; however, the services do not have to be funded at their current levels.

Financing Medical Education

PPS support of direct and indirect medical education is separate from its payments for patient care. The separation of medical education and patient care costs results from a recognition that teaching hospitals are more costly than other hospitals and should be explicitly reimbursed for their educational costs. Medicare made this decision based upon a statistical analysis that determined the incremental cost of clinical training programs (Pettingill and Vertrees 1982). Considerable additional research has attempted to refine the empirical estimates of the cost of training residents, nurses, and allied health professionals (Anderson and Lave 1986; Cameron 1985; Commonwealth Fund Task Force 1985; Arthur Young 1986). At the present time, however, there is no consensus concerning the incremental cost of operating these programs. Education and patient care are frequently performed simultaneously, so any separation of these costs is somewhat arbitrary.

One position is that educational costs should be financed from governmental resources other than Medicare (Congress, Social Security Advisory Council 1984). The basic argument is that resources collected for patient care services should not be used to finance clinical education. This argument, however, does not recognize the inextricable relationship between production of education and patient care, nor does it recognize that the cost of on-the-job training is incorporated in the cost of production in most industries (Commonwealth Fund Task Force 1985).

Equally important is the debate over what type of training should be sponsored. Policy analysts have questioned whether public funds should support only specific residency programs based on societal needs. Some have argued that public funds should not finance training in specialties in which a surplus is anticipated (Commonwealth Fund Task Force 1985; Petersdorf 1985).

One alternative would be to discontinue direct funding of resident training through hospitals; instead, residency programs could be permitted to bill payers for the services provided by residents. Under this system, many residents could generate patient care revenues sufficient to cover the cost of their training (Anderson and Lave 1986). This approach to financing training is similar to the manner in which training of other professionals who have finished their formal academic work is supported. Federal funding could still be provided for certain residency programs in specialties that are deemed to be in short supply or are not financially self-supporting. Grants could be made to hospitals, health maintenance organizations, or other institutions to encourage them to establish residency programs that are in the public interest.

Unsponsored Research and Technological Innovation

Unsponsored research and technological innovation are particularly vulnerable under PPS because unlike medical education, these products have not been supported through an explicit payment in PPS. Historically, most unsponsored research, technological innovation, and even a portion of the sponsored research have been financed from patient care revenues (Commonwealth Fund Task Force 1985). The current price-competitive environment will retard the development of these products unless financial support for their development is provided.

If society wants to maintain the current level of biomedical research and medical innovation, it must increase the level of direct appropriations for these services. Policymakers could increase the DRG payment rate to hospitals that perform research and technological development. This adjustment would be similar to the PPS adjustment for indirect medical education costs and could be based upon the number or volume of National Institutes of Health (NIH) grants received. Alternatively, Congress could increase the number and size of NIH grants for clinical research or include an indirect cost allowance for pilot research projects and research development. In addition, teaching hospitals should be encouraged to assess carefully the indirect costs of sponsored biomedical research and to include all indirect costs in submissions to NIH, private industry, foundations, and other funding sources. Most hospitals do not know how much biomedical research adds to the cost of the hospital. Without that information it is impossible to determine whether research is self-supporting.

Capital

The original PPS legislation required the Secretary of Health and Human Services to submit a report to Congress recommending a method for incorporating capital into PPS. The statute mandated that this report should review the issues associated with capital payment policy. Congress was unwilling to incorporate capital into the original PPS legislation because of the complexity of issues involved. Instead, Congress has opted to postpone the decision until 1991 and to pay hospitals a portion of their capital costs.

In general, capital payment reform is necessary because of the perverse incentives created by cost-based reimbursement for capital (Anderson and Ginsburg 1983). Under cost-based reimbursement, hospitals receive a payment for depreciation, interest, and rent expenses associated with the percentage of Medicare patients treated. Hospitals are therefore insensitive to changes in interest rates and protected from the risks inherent in investing in capital. A goal of any capital payment reform is to encourage hospitals to invest more prudently than they did in the past. However, the passage of PPS created more perverse incentives. The combination of prospective payment for operating costs and cost-based reimbursement for capital costs created incentives for hospitals to substitute capital for labor (Anderson and Ginsburg 1984). Development of a prospective payment system for capital would eliminate this incentive. Various options for incorporating capital into PPS have been explored for several years. In general, the debate on capital policy centers on three topics: (1) the aggregate level of capital payment; (2) the method of allocating payment to individual hospitals; and (3) methods of phasing in any new system.

The Aggregate Level of Capital Payment

Arguments have been presented both for paying more and for paying less than Medicare pays currently for capital. Probably the best argument for paying more is that the current method of paying for capital—historical cost depreciation—does not adjust for inflation once the capital is purchased. As a result, hospitals are unable to replace capital after it has depreciated because inflation has substantially raised the cost of the replacement equipment. One argument that supports lower Medicare payment for capital (aside from obligatory federal budgetary arguments) is that occupancy rates are declining and thus less capital may be necessary in the future (Anderson and Ginsburg 1984).

Several analysts have made empirical estimates of the future capital requirements of the hospital industry (Cohodes 1983; Cohodes and Kinkead 1984). Numerical estimates of the need for capital can vary widely depending on the assumptions and measure of need. Estimates of total hospital capital need in the 1980s varied from $49 billion to $231 billion (Anderson and Ginsburg 1984). Many have argued that given the difficulty of measuring need and the wide variation among empirical estimates of need, the current level of spending (adjusted for inflation) should be continued. This policy would result in the expenditure of $100 billion on capital during the 1980s. This proposal is budget neutral in the sense that the aggregate level of Medicare capital expenditures is not changed by this proposal. As a result, the historical relationship between capital and operating cost would remain unchanged.

The Method of Allocating Capital Funds

Much of the debate about capital concerns the method of allocating capital payments to individual hospitals. Hospitals spend an average of approximately 9 percent of their budget on capital. The current distribution of capital resources is relatively uniform across hospital groups (Anderson 1986), although there are individual hospitals at each extreme. Teaching and public hospitals spend less than 9 percent, while for-profit hospitals spend more. Most of the discussion about allocation of Medicare's capital dollars, therefore, concerns the needs of individual hospitals with specific problems rather than specific groups of hospitals.

The two primary alternatives for allocating capital among hospitals are either adopting a new prospective payment system for capital or modifying the existing cost-based reimbursement system. Cost-based reimbursement for capital could continue, with some overall limit on spending. Suggested modifications include placing upper limits on capital expenditures on either a per-bed or peradmission basis or using the planning process to enforce statewide limits on total capital expenditures. The prospective payment option would combine operating and capital payments into a single DRG payment (Anderson and Ginsburg 1983). This proposal would put hospitals entirely at risk for their capital costs, offering incentives to economize in both purchasing and financing decisions.

Our review of the various proposals and the incentives created by each suggests that a single payment incorporating capital and operating expenditures is the most logical. This permits the hospital to choose the most appropriate combination of inputs to produce hospital care. It recognizes that capital and labor are both necessary to produce hospital care and allows the hospital administrator to determine the optimal mix of capital and operating expenditures.

The Transition Period

Given the long life of many capital assets and the difficulty of renegotiating capital payment arrangements, the difficulties of moving from a cost-based to a prospective payment system are much greater for capital than for operating costs. Hospitals that have recently expanded or renovated may have significant financial obligations for many years. These obligations are frequently scheduled to be paid off at a fixed rate. Any abrupt transition to a prospective payment system that did not recognize recent commitments could seriously jeopardize a hospital's ability to repay its loans.

For this reason, it may be necessary to phase in a prospective payment system for capital. To balance the needs of hospitals in different stages of their capital cycles, it may be necessary to give higher payments to hospitals that have just had a major capital project than to hospitals that have not invested recently. Providing too much to those hospitals that have expanded recently, however, will not provide adequate funds for hospitals to acquire capital in the future. One option is to pay hospitals a blend of the amount to which they would be entitled under the old, cost-based reimbursement system and what they would receive under the new, prospective system. Such a blend could be paid over a period of several years, with the cost-based proportion representing an increasingly smaller portion of the payment and the prospective payment portion an increasingly larger proportion. This policy can be justified by research that demonstrates that the effect of a major capital project on total costs generally is absorbed by a hospital after seven years (Krystenak 1983).

Controlling Admissions

Traditionally, hospitals have responded to price controls either by increasing the number of visits or by increasing the quantity of services provided per encounter (Aaron 1984). Total revenue is equal to price times quantity, and when price is constrained, total revenue can be increased only by increasing quantity.

Under PPS, it was expected that admission rates would rise, because to generate revenues under PPS, hospitals could increase revenues by raising the admission rate. In addition, the recent decline in hospital occupancy rates has created incentives for hospital administrators to fill beds. PPS offers other incentives for hospitals to increase admissions (Anderson and Steinberg 1984b). Most economists estimate that the marginal cost of a hospital admission is approximately 60 percent of the average cost (Lipscomb, Raskin, and Eichenholz 1978). When the PPS rates were first established, they were equal to the average cost of treating a patient within the DRG. Hospitals have an economic incentive to increase the number of admissions because the marginal cost is substantially less than the average cost.

There are incentives for the hospital to increase readmissions. For each admission the hospital receives one payment, which, aside from additional payments for complications or comorbidities, creates disincentives to treat patients with multiple problems during one admission. The economic incentive is to treat one of the diagnoses, discharge the patient, and then readmit the patient for the second diagnosis (Anderson and Steinberg 1984a). Readmissions may also occur as a result of economic pressures to discharge a patient prematurely. DRG payments are fixed regardless of length of stay (aside from outliers); thus hospitals have an incentive to reduce lengths of stay. It has been suggested that early discharge could result in complications or cause a physician to overlook certain comorbidities, resulting in an increase in the readmission rate.

Admission rates are difficult to regulate because so little is known about the decision to admit a patient to a hospital. Research suggests that the "medical practice factor" is a much better predictor of general hospitalization rates in a community than either demographic factors or self-reported health status (Wennberg 1984). Analysis of hospitalization rates among the Medicare population shows significant variations across regions of the country and even within small geographic areas (Wennberg 1986). Similar variations in hospital readmission rates have also been found (Gornick, Newton, and Hackerman 1980). Until more is known about why a specific person is admitted or why there is variation among geographic regions, it will be difficult to regulate admission rates.

Two general strategies have been employed to control admission rates in the past. Neither has been particularly effective. One approach has been to adjust the payment formula to control admission rates. This strategy is based on the knowledge that the marginal cost of an admission is less than the average cost. Under an "admission load adjustment," a hospital's payment decreases when admissions increase, and the payment increases when admission rates decline. This formula was used in Nixon's Economic Stabilization Program.

There are a number of problems with this formula approach. First, although marginal costs are generally assumed to be 60 percent of average costs, this estimate is based on certain assumptions about the length of time a hospital has to respond to the change in admissions, whether the change in admissions was anticipated, and what kinds of cases were represented in the increased admissions rate. As a result, empirical estimates of the marginal cost may vary from 10 percent to 90 percent of average costs, depending on these factors (Lipscomb, Raskin, and Eichenholz 1978). A second problem with this approach is that it is inconsistent with the basic tenets of prospective payment. A fundamental tenet of PPS is that all hospitals within a community should be paid the same for treating an identical patient, and adjusting the payment level based upon changes in admission rates would violate this principle.

A second approach to controlling admissions has been to monitor admission rates by reviewing individual cases. The Medicare program has chosen this approach to control admission rates under PPS. PROs were created in each state to monitor admissions under PPS. The PRO is generally an organization comprised of physicians that contracts with the federal government to monitor other physicians in the state. The PRO reviews individual cases as well as admission patterns on both the physician and the hospital level to see whether the admissions are appropriate. In addition, PROs review all readmissions within a specified period and outlier cases. Despite all of the incentives for hospitals to increase admissions under PPS, the failure to observe this increase may be attributable to PRO review efforts.

The underlying tenets of the PRO program, however, make it difficult for the program to be effective over the longer term. The PRO program is organized so that physicians monitor physicians, a classic example of the regulated controlling the regulators. It is unclear what real incentives physicians have to monitor other physicians. A second problem with the PRO program is that standards are set on a state-by-state basis. Given the wide variation in admission rates by geographic location (Wennberg 1984) and the PRO's emphasis on local practice, it is not likely that PROs will be effective in reducing the geographic variation of hospital admissions. A third problem is that standards of comparison for admission do not exist. Each PRO—and ultimately each physician—can argue that any admission is medically necessary. Without standards it is difficult to prove otherwise. Finally, this type of regulation is extremely expensive because it requires review of individual cases. Rather than creating financial incentives for physicians to behave appropriately, this regulation imposes sanctions for inappropriate behavior.

Conclusion and Recommendations

Modifying the Medicare PPS

The Medicare PPS has been implemented and is working to encourage hospitals to reduce the length of patient stays. However, it is incomplete in many respects and could have adverse effects over the intermediate term on many aspects of hospital care. The following changes are recommended to make intermediate improvements in the system:

- A formula for establishing increases in PPS rates over a longer time period will promote predictability in hospital rates.
- Incorporation of an adjustment to the DRG system for the complexity of cases treated will more appropriately reimburse hospitals for very expensive patients.
- Adjustments to the PPS rates for inner city location and nonlabor costs will make the system more equitable.
- Making refinements to the method of financing medical education, biomedical research, and technological change will promote the type of services that society wants to have hospitals produce.

• Incorporating capital into PPS will remove the perverse incentives to overinvest in capital.

These are only short-term solutions. PPS probably can never be designed so that each hospital receives exactly the right level of payment for each patient. There are too many factors determining why one patient or one hospital is more expensive than another. No payment formula can ever adjust for all these factors without becoming prohibitively complex.

Determining the appropriate level of payment for each patient is important, however, because if hospitals can determine that they can make a profit on one patient and lose money on another patient, then there are economic incentives to discriminate against the unprofitable patient. PPS was based on the assumption that hospitals would be willing to make money on some patients, lose money on others, and still show a profit. Unfortunately many hospital administrators have concentrated their monitoring efforts on patients who stay longer than average or cost more than average. As hospital administrators gain further experience, there is every reason to believe that they will try to avoid those patients that are relatively less profitable.

A second fundamental problem with PPS is that there is an economic incentive to increase admission rates. This incentive is quite powerful, although it has not been manifest during the early years of PPS. If at some time the number of admissions increases, there is no control mechanism built into PPS. The best solution, therefore, would be to rely on other utilization control measures or to move to a capitation system, which would introduce incentives to control the admission rate.

An All-Payer PPS

A major difficulty with the Medicare PPS over the longer term is that the average Medicare payment rates are unlikely to keep pace with those for privately insured patients. This is true due to strong political incentives to limit increases in Medicare payment rates, while payment rates of privately insured patients are unregulated and are not subject to any coordinated policy. If, as might be anticipated, hospital costs resume a rapid inflationary pace, Medicare and private payment rates will diverge rapidly.

It is this divergence that all-payer systems seek to avoid. Once two levels of payment are established, it is politically difficult to bring them into balance. Lowering private rates to the Medicare level would result in a dramatic loss of revenues to hospitals; raising Medicare payment rates to private rates would result in a dramatic increase in governmental outlays. Neither option is politically attractive.

Yet, as the gap between Medicare and privately insured patients widens, certain consequences become more likely. Some hospitals may be unwilling to accept Medicare patients and will specialize on care of the nonelderly. Others will reduce the quality and amenities of care available to Medicare patients and maintain a different standard of care for privately insured patients. In addition, the rapid increase in the uncontrolled cost of privately insured patients will lead to rapid increases in employer-paid private health insurance premiums. Employers may seek to protect themselves by capping their contributions to employee health insurance plans, leaving employees to bear the brunt of rapid escalation in costs. In either case pressure will begin to build for an effective health care cost containment policy that will address overall inflation in health care costs.

One option would be to extend PPS to privately insured patients and to all Medicaid programs. A number of technical issues would need to be resolved to make such an approach feasible. A major issue is the availability of data to calculate weights and standard payment amounts. The standard payment amounts and DRG weights used by Medicare were calculated using a national sample of elderly Medicare patient records. No equivalent data set exists for patients of all ages; however, policymakers might consider using data from state governments in order to calculate rational rates and payment amounts. Several states have such data. The billing data provided by these authorities would be useful to federal policymakers for this purpose.

A second issue is whether under a national all-payer PPS all payers would pay identical rates. One alternative would be to use a common set of standard payment amounts and weights for all payers. Another option would be to use a different set of prices (i.e., standard payment amounts) for each payer. This approach would account for the variation in costs that is attributable to the variation in the mix of patients insured by different payers. For example, the cost of bypass surgery for Medicare patients may be different from that of patients insured by Blue Cross because of the difference in the ages of those patients. Using separate standard payment amounts that are essentially averages for the insured group would capture this variation.

A third issue is what costs should be included in the standard payment amount. Medicare's standard payment amounts exclude the bad debt of any patients not insured by Medicare; however, several all-payer systems explicitly include bad debt and charity care in the calculation of prices. These costs are considered legitimate costs of doing business.

Given these difficult issues, it is important that research continue not only to evaluate the impact of the Medicare PPS but also to support the development of modifications to improve the system and to extend it more broadly to other payers.

Chapter 4

Medicaid: State Approaches to
Cost Containment for the Poor

Medicaid plays a key role in financing health care for America's poor, paying for hospital and physician care for approximately one out of every ten Americans each year. Although Medicaid provides financial assistance with medical bills to 24 million poor Americans, it is not immune to budget pressures and constraints. Medicaid is a public program dependent on federal and state tax dollars to finance health care. When fiscal pressures increase at the federal or state level, Medicaid is often a primary target for budget cuts.

The pressure to cut Medicaid spending became especially strong in 1981, when the Reagan administration took office with a public mandate to decrease taxes and cut federal nondefense domestic spending (Blendon and Moloney 1982). In response to reduced federal support for Medicaid and other domestic programs, as well as their own economic and budgetary problems, many states cut back or altered their Medicaid program. Many states accomplished savings by instituting changes in provider payment levels and methods.

This chapter describes the cost containment approaches employed by the states in their Medicaid programs in response to the fiscal pressures of the 1980s. The first section discusses Medicaid's role as a payer of hospital and health care for the poor. The second section reviews changes in Medicaid policy at the federal level since 1980, and the third section describes state Medicaid policy responses. The fourth section provides a case study of Wisconsin's innovative approach to health care delivery reform using case management and prepaid capitated care. The final section discusses the policy implications of provider payment reform under state Medicaid programs.

Medicaid as a Payer of Health Services for the Poor

Medicaid is a joint federal-state program under which the states provide medical benefits to low-income individuals who meet categorical criteria and income and assets requirements. Medicaid eligibility primarily follows the categorical criteria for welfare assistance—the elderly, the disabled, and children from single-parent families and their parents. States are required to extend Medicaid coverage to all recipients of cash assistance under Aid to Families with Dependent Children (AFDC) and to most elderly and disabled who receive cash assistance from the Supplemental Security Income (SSI) program.

States have the most discretion in terms of eligibility and income standards for poor children and families and often limit the extent of coverage for this group. Many poor families are not covered because state income standards for AFDC and Medicaid eligibility are well below the poverty level. Many states do not extend coverage to two-parent families or to medically needy individuals who are impoverished by large medical expenses.

Medicaid coverage of the aged, the blind, and the disabled is more consistent nationally than coverage of poor children because the SSI cash assistance program has uniform national eligibility criteria, leaving states with less discretion. Aged, blind, and disabled Medicaid beneficiaries are also generally eligible for care under Medicare and primarily use Medicaid to supplement acute-care services financed by Medicare and to pay for long-term care. All states cover hospital and physician services, but coverage of other services varies widely. Payment levels and utilization controls on hospital and physician care also vary among states, making the scope of Medicaid benefits far from uniform in the various states. As a result, Medicaid neither covers all the poor nor provides those who are covered with comprehensive benefits.

Medicaid's original goal was to encourage states to provide comprehensive health care coverage to the nation's poor (Davis and Schoen 1978). From enactment in 1965 to 1971, expenditures grew rapidly from $1.6 billion to $6.3 billion, as states initiated their programs and expanded coverage. The 1972 amendments to the Social Security Act provided the first major changes in the direction of Medicaid coverage. In response to some states' concern about the growing cost of the program, the goal of comprehensive coverage of the poor by Medicaid was eliminated. However, coverage of the aged, the blind, and the disabled was expanded as Medicaid coverage was extended to most beneficiaries of the new SSI federal cash assistance program. In addition, intermediate care facilities for the mentally retarded were added as a benefit, expanding coverage for that population. As a result, Medicaid spending increased at an annual rate of 25 percent from 1971 to 1975 (HCFA 1986a).

By 1976 the Medicaid program had 22.9 million beneficiaries and expenditures of $14.1 billion (HCFA 1986a). The years from 1976 to 1980 saw two major trends in Medicaid, a decline in program eligibility and a rapid increase in spending due to inflation. The decline in eligibility was partially a result of states' failure to index income eligibility standards to inflation. By 1980 the number of people eligible for Medicaid had dropped to 21.6 million, but spending had increased to $23.3 billion. Rising prices and increased intensity of medical services accounted for almost all of the increase in Medicaid spending during this period.

Beginning in 1980 and continuing through today, Medicaid has been in a period of fiscal retrenchment. Despite the economic recession in 1981 and the high levels of unemployment, as well as the increased number of people living in poverty, the number of people covered by Medicaid did not increase. From 1980 to 1985 Medicaid eligibility increased only modestly from 21.6 million to 21.7 million beneficiaries, but expenditures grew from $23.3 billion in 1980 to $37.5 billion in 1985. The annual rate of increase in Medicaid expenditures during this period was 8 percent. Price increases accounted for a 10 percent annual rate of increase, but expenditures were moderated by a 2 percent decrease in Medicaid utilization (Muse 1987). Since 1985, expansions in Medicaid coverage have increased the number of Medicaid beneficiaries from 21.7 million to 24.2 million in 1988. Medicaid program costs are estimated to increase to 55.1 billion for 1988 (House Committee on Ways and Means 1988).

New Federal Policy Directions for Medicaid, 1980–1984

By 1980, inflation and cost containment had become the dominant concerns in the health care system as well as in the national economy. Double-digit inflation, high rates of unemployment, and growing concern over increasing taxes to reduce the federal deficit combined to focus public attention on the economy. In the midst of a serious recession in 1981, action to strengthen the economy and reduce inflation was a priority for public policy.

With Reagan's election in the fall of 1980 a new plan for national economic recovery calling for reduced federal domestic spending, substantial increases in military spending, and cuts in federal taxes to stimulate economic growth was proposed. As part of this reordering, Medicaid was among the social welfare programs targeted for major cuts and restructuring (Rowland, Lyons, and Edwards 1988).

The first Reagan budget, submitted to Congress in 1981, proposed to cap federal spending for Medicaid. Medicaid is an open-ended entitlement program under which states pay for health care services on behalf of eligible beneficiaries. The federal government matches state spending, with no upper limit on the amount it will match. The Reagan administration proposal would have ended the entitlement nature of Medicaid by placing an upper limit or "cap" on what the federal government would spend on Medicaid in any given year. State expenditures would have been matched only up to the federal maximum. Once that fixed amount was reached, the states would have been faced with the choice of cutting their Medicaid spending to stay within the federal limits or paying for the additional spending solely with state funds. If implemented, this cap would have resulted in an estimated cut of $9 billion in federal Medicaid spending from 1981 to 1985 (Iglehart 1985a).

Congress did not enact the Medicaid cap proposal. Strong opposition from the states as well as from advocates of the poor and health care providers saved the entitlement nature of Medicaid. The states were concerned that a ceiling on federal spending would result in pressure for additional spending of state dollars to compensate for federal reductions. Advocates were concerned that a spending ceiling would limit the scope of program coverage and lead to an erosion in benefits and eligibility. Both parties argued that the Reagan administration's proposed cap represented an abandonment of the federal government's commitment to help finance health care for the poor. Their arguments ultimately persuaded Congress to retain the existing structure of Medicaid.

The drive to cut federal spending meant, however, that although the structure of Medicaid was preserved, Medicaid was not protected from large spending cuts. The Omnibus Budget Reconciliation Act of 1981 (OBRA) imposed a temporary reduction in the federal share of Medicaid spending in each state of up to 3 percent in 1982. In 1983 the reduction level increased to 4 percent, and in 1984 to 4.5 percent. States were able to offset some of the reductions by meeting quantitative targets for cost containment or having an all-payer rate-setting program. It is estimated that these reductions cut federal Medicaid spending by over $4 billion from 1980 through 1984 (House Committee on Energy and Commerce 1986).

Along with the reduced federal aid, the OBRA legislation gave states greater flexibility with regard to the scope and design of their Medicaid programs in order to provide additional options to reduce program spending. Much of this new authority concerned state discretion with regard to provider payment and ability to restrict the use of services by beneficiaries. Specifically, the OBRA legislation gave states new authority over hospital payment under Medicaid and allowed states to experiment with alternative delivery systems as a means of restructuring care to reduce expenditures.

Before 1981 states had been required to pay hospitals using the Medicare principles of hospital payment (see chapter 2). States were allowed to apply for permission to use alternative payment systems, but since the process was cumbersome, few states implemented alternative systems. The states seeking alternative system approval tended to be the states with all-payer rate setting that wanted to include Medicaid in their across-the-board systems. With OBRA, states gained the authority to determine Medicaid hospital payment methods and levels. In addition, they gained new authority to experiment with alternatives to fee-for-service payment for physicians involving case management, capitated payment, and limitations on freedom of choice of physicians or other health care providers. With the new authority, states could design prepaid enrollment systems for the poor without being constrained by the requirements associated with federally qualified HMOs.

After OBRA, Medicaid continued to be a target for restructuring and deep cuts in each of the Reagan budgets. After 1981, however, Congress protected the program from major cutbacks and did not extend the temporary reductions in the federal share after they expired in 1984. Thus, by 1984, federal program financing had been restored.

Despite pressure to restrain spending, in both 1984 and 1985 Congress actually expanded Medicaid coverage by requiring states to cover all pregnant women and children eligible under state income standards under their programs. In 1986 Congress made federal Medicaid matching funds available if states, at their option, expanded coverage to pregnant women and young children or elderly and disabled individuals with incomes up to the federal poverty level. In 1987 Congress included provisions in OBRA that permit states to increase coverage for pregnant women and infants up to 185 percent of the poverty level. The Medicare Catastrophic Coverage Act of 1988 further expands Medicaid by requiring state Medicaid programs to pay the Medicare premium, copayment, and drug benefit for Medicare beneficiaries with an income below the poverty line. States are also required to provide pregnancy services to pregnant women with an income below the poverty line and full Medicaid benefits to poor children under age one.

In sum, the basic purpose and structure of Medicaid as an entitlement program was retained, but federal budgetary pressure required savings from Medicaid as part of each year's congressional budget reconciliation process. As a result of the over $4 billion in federal spending cuts, states were given additional discretion over eligibility and benefits, Medicaid hospital payment rates were decoupled from Medicare, and states were permitted to limit beneficiaries' choice of providers (House Committee on Energy and Commerce 1986). The impact of these federal policy changes on Medicaid beneficiaries and providers thus depended on the policy choices made by each state.

State Medicaid Policy Responses

The Medicaid programs in the various states have undergone significant changes in response to the federal financing cutbacks, as well as state fiscal problems (Bovbjerg and Holahan 1982; Feder and Holahan 1985). With the enactment of OBRA, states had to accept a temporary reduction in federal financial support as the price for greater flexibility with regard to program design. Many responded to the federal reductions by enacting cuts in their programs instead of making up the difference with state revenues.

Restrictions in eligibility and benefits are, on the surface, a direct and easily designed method to reduce state expenditures under Medicaid. Limits on income eligibility standards, coverage of optional groups, and amount of covered services are familiar strategies to states seeking to constrain costs. Most states turned to these familiar techniques when fiscal pressures and federal cutbacks made reduced spending a top priority in 1981. However, many states also turned to new ways to pay for hospital care and alternative delivery systems to supplement the savings that could be achieved from direct cuts in eligibility and benefits.

Changes in the Scope of Medicaid Coverage of the Poor

During the period 1980–84, eligibility for Medicaid was directly or indirectly limited for children and families in most states because of federal and state changes in AFDC program cash assistance eligibility policy or Medicaid policy. As a result of these changes, Medicaid coverage of the poor and near poor population declined from 53 percent in 1980 to 46 percent in 1985 (Blendon 1986a). The major contributors to this decline were failure to update state income standards, changes in welfare policy as a result of OBRA, and direct Medicaid eligibility changes.

Nationwide, the state Medicaid income eligibility standards as a percentage of the poverty level dropped from 55 percent in 1980 to 47 percent in 1984 (see table 4.1). In essence, this lowering of the Medicaid eligibility standards means that a smaller proportion of poor people were covered by Medicaid in 1984 than in 1980. By 1986, however, this downward trend had reversed. Although still below the 1980 level, Medicaid income eligibility levels had increased to 51 percent of poverty.

The proportion of poor people covered by Medicaid also declined because of changes in federal welfare policy. OBRA established new limits on both income and resources for AFDC and Medicaid eligibility. The OBRA welfare changes limited state flexibility, especially with regard to working families, and eliminated state discretion over asset standards for AFDC and Medicaid eligibility. Under the new, uniform rules, families are allowed to possess a home of any value but only one automobile

Table 4.1. Medicaid Eligibility Standards: AFDC Payment Standard or Medically Needy Standard for a Family of Four and Standard as a Percentage of Poverty, 1980, 1984, and 1986

	1980		1984		1986	
State[a]	Eligibility Standard	Eligibility Standard as Percentage of Poverty	Eligibility Standard	Eligibility Standard as Percentage of Poverty	Eligibility Standard	Eligibility Standard as Percentage of Poverty
Federal poverty level, family of 4	$8,414	100	$10,610	100	$11,203	100
Average	$4,593	55	$ 4,992	47	$ 5,665	51
Alabama	1,776	21	1,764	17	1,764	16
Alaska	6,168	73	9,300	88	9,300	83
Arkansas*	3,100	37	3,096	29	3,600	32
California*	7,800	93	9,612	91	11,208	100
Colorado	4,212	50	4,896	46	4,332	39
Connecticut*	6,204	74	7,500	71	9,600	86
Delaware	3,744	44	4,032	38	4,188	37
District of Columbia*	4,864	58	4,392	41	4,788	43
Florida	2,760	33	3,276	31	3,576	32
Georgia	2,316	28	2,856	27	4,296	38
Hawaii*	6,600	78	6,600	62	6,600	59
Idaho	4,404	52	3,648	34	3,648	33
Illinois*	4,200	50	4,416	42	6,204	55
Indiana	3,780	45	3,924	37	4,356	39
Iowa	5,028	60	5,028	47	6,096	54
Kansas*	4,920	58	5,160	49	5,520	49
Kentucky*	3,800	45	3,804	36	3,804	34
Louisiana*	3,504	42	3,804	36	3,804	34
Maine*	5,700	68	5,196	49	7,896	70
Maryland*	4,104	49	4,704	44	4,740	42
Massachusetts*	5,280	63	5,340	50	6,108	55
Michigan*	5,992	71	5,904	56	6,960	62
Minnesota*	5,832	69	6,996	66	7,392	66
Mississippi	3,024	36	3,924	37	3,924	35
Missouri	3,480	41	3,660	34	3,660	33
Montana*	5,304	63	5,100	48	5,112	46
Nebraska*	5,600	67	6,300	59	6,300	56
Nevada	3,768	45	3,264	31	4,092	37
New Hampshire*	4,704	56	4,920	46	5,700	51
New Jersey	4,968	59	4,968	47	5,580	50

Table 4.1. Continued

State[a]	1980		1984		1986	
	Eligibility Standard	Eligibility Standard as Percentage of Poverty	Eligibility Standard	Eligibility Standard as Percentage of Poverty	Eligibility Standard	Eligibility Standard as Percentage of Poverty
New Mexico	3,204	38	2,496	24	2,496	22
New York*	5,712	68	7,224	68	8,484	76
North Carolina*	3,400	40	3,600	34	4,404	39
North Dakota*	6,360	76	6,360	60	6,360	57
Ohio	3,924	47	4,116	39	4,488	40
Oklahoma*	5,600	67	5,604	53	6,204	55
Oregon*	5,292	63	5,352	50	7,716	69
Pennsylvania*	4,750	56	5,496	52	5,496	49
Rhode Island*	6,900	82	7,200	68	7,296	65
South Carolina	1,896	23	2,088	20	2,868	26
South Dakota	4,332	51	4,332	41	4,452	40
Tennessee*	2,400	29	2,460	23	3,000	27
Texas	1,680	20	2,136	20	3,612	32
Utah*	5,832	69	6,648	63	7,020	63
Vermont*	6,624	79	7,464	70	7,476	67
Virginia*	4,020	48	4,404	42	13,200	118
Washington*	6,432	76	6,372	60	6,936	62
West Virginia*	3,300	39	5,976	56	3,744	33
Wisconsin*	7,000	83	8,640	81	9,168	82
Wyoming	4,080	48	4,260	40	4,680	42

Sources: House Committee on Ways and Means 1987; HCFA 1982, 1985, 1987a.
Note: In states with a Medically Needy Program, the Medically Needy payment standard is used to determine eligibility when it is higher than the AFDC payment standard.
[a]An asterisk indicates that the state has a Medically Needy Program.

worth up to $1,500 and other personal property up to $1,000 (Hill 1984).

OBRA also limited eligibility for cash assistance and Medicaid for certain groups of potential beneficiaries. Cash assistance to first-time pregnant women with no other children was prohibited before the sixth month of pregnancy. Medicaid coverage of children aged eighteen to twenty-one was made optional, and states were permitted to vary income and assets eligibility levels among the medically needy. Despite the pressure to cut program spending, Congress sought to expand coverage of poor pregnant women and infants under Medicaid and eliminated some state discretion over eligibility in the 1984 and 1985 budget reconciliation legislative packages. In response to growing concern about high levels of infant mortality among the poor, expansions of Medicaid coverage for pregnant women and children in two-parent families were enacted as mandatory provisions.

In summary, the eligibility picture was mixed over the Reagan years. The 1981–82 period clearly marked a reduction in Medicaid eligibility for children and their families, largely driven by cutbacks in the AFDC program. However, by 1984 the pendulum had swung back, and Medicaid care for pregnant women and children had returned to the legislative agenda. In 1988 Congress enacted legislation requiring states to cover all pregnant women and infants in single- or two-parent families up to the federal poverty level and giving them the option of extending coverage to 185 percent of poverty.

The scope of Medicaid coverage of the poverty population has important implications for providers. The poor without Medicaid coverage are often uninsured for their medical expenses (Davis and Rowland 1983). As a result of restrictions in Medicaid eligibility, hospitals and other providers are likely to experience an increase in the proportion of poor people seeking treatment who are uninsured and an associated increase in bad debts.

Limits on Medicaid Benefits as a Cost Containment Measure

For poor children and their families, Medicaid provides for most acute health care as well as long-term care services, when needed. States have substantial freedom to determine the range and level of benefits, but they are required to cover inpatient and outpatient hospital services, physician services, laboratory and x-ray services, family planning, screening and diagnostic services for children, and home health and nursing home care in skilled nursing facilities for adults. States can elect to provide other services, including prescription drugs, dental care, and nursing home care in intermediate care facilities.

States can restrict the use of required and optional benefits by limiting the number of physician visits or the number of days of hospital care or by imposing utilization controls or nominal copayments. Prior to the OBRA legislation, restrictions on benefits were the major means by which states tried to limit Medicaid utilization and costs. During the 1980–85 period, states continued to utilize benefit restrictions to restrain costs but now coupled these restrictions with payment limits on providers and new delivery mechanisms, as discussed in the next sections.

For hospital care, states can employ two types of benefit limitations: (1) a limit on the number of days of hospital care covered per admission or per year and (2) a requirement for prior authorization for specific procedures or elective surgery. As shown in table 4.2, the number of states imposing day limits has declined from eighteen in 1980 to eleven in 1986. Prior authorization is a more popular approach: twenty-two states

Table 4.2. Restrictions on Hospital Benefits, 1980, 1984, and 1986

State	Limits on Hospital Days per Admission or per Year			Preauthorization Required			Other Controls		
	1980	1984	1986	1980	1984	1986	1980	1984	1986
Total Number	18	15	11	12	21	22	14	39	43
Alabama	15/yr	12/yr	12/yr		X	X	X	X	X
Alaska				X	X				X
Arizona[a]									
Arkansas	26/yr		35/yr			X		X	X
California				X	X	X	X'	X	X
Colorado								X	X
Connecticut								X	X
Delaware									X
District of Columbia				X	X			X	X
Florida	45/yr	45/yr	45/yr					X	X
Georgia				X	X	X		X	X
Hawaii	8/ad			X				X	X
Idaho	40/ad	40/yr	40/yr				X		
Illinois	45/yr							X	X
Indiana					X	X		X	
Iowa					X	X		X	X
Kansas				X			X	X	X
Kentucky	21/ad	14/ad	14/ad		X		X	X	X
Louisiana	15/yr					X		X	X
Maine		30/yr		X				X	
Maryland		20/ad		X	X	X		X	X
Massachusetts							X		
Michigan				X	X	X		X	X
Minnesota				X	X			X	X
Mississippi	20/yr	20/yr	15/yr					X	X
Missouri	21/ad							X	X
Montana									X
Nebraska				X				X	X
Nevada							X	X	X
New Hampshire				X			X		X
New Jersey				X	X	X	X	X	X
New Mexico				X	X			X	X
New York						X		X	X
North Carolina				X	X	X	X	X	X
North Dakota									

Table 4.2. Continued

State	Limits on Hospital Days per Admission or per Year			Preauthorization Required			Other Controls		
	1980	1984	1986	1980	1984	1986	1980	1984	1986
Ohio	60/ad	30/ad				X		X	X
Oklahoma	10/ad	10/ad						X	X
Oregon	21/yr	18/yr	18/yr	X					X
Pennsylvania							X	X	X
Rhode Island				X	X	X		X	X
South Carolina		12/yr		X	X	X	X	X	X
South Dakota	60/yr								
Tennessee	20/yr	14/yr	14/yr					X	X
Texas	30/ad	30/ad	30/ad					X	X
Utah					X	X		X	X
Vermont					X	X		X	X
Virginia	14/ad	21/ad	21/yr					X	X
Washington						X	X	X	X
West Virginia	60/yr	20/yr	60/yr						
Wisconsin				X	X	X			X
Wyoming								X	X

Sources: HCFA 1982, 1985, 1987a.
[a]Arizona had no program in these years.

now impose such a limit, compared with twelve states in 1980. From 1980 to 1986 the number of states imposing some limit on the range of services that can be provided and the locational setting increased from fourteen to forty-three. In 1986 only four states (Maine, Massachusetts, North Dakota, and South Dakota) were without any inpatient hospital utilization controls (HCFA 1987a).

Limitations on physician services are also a common state cost containment strategy. Physicians' services have been limited by either the number of visits or types of procedures that can be performed in all but seven states. In addition, in 1986 eleven states limited the number of visits to hospital outpatient departments and fourteen states limited coverage to specific procedures, excluding routine physical examinations or experimental procedures. Prior authorization is required for certain other services and/or procedures in fourteen states as a further attempt to control utilization (HCFA 1987a).

Limits on covered days of service mean that when hospitals treat Medicaid patients, the full cost of care may not be recovered if the patient's care requirements exceed the limits of Medicaid coverage. The care exceeding Medicaid coverage would become uncompensated care and would be counted as bad debts or charity care.

New Systems for Medicaid Hospital Payment

The most direct mechanism to reduce Medicaid spending for hospital care is to limit the amount hospitals are paid for care to Medicaid beneficiaries. However, from the enactment of Medicaid in 1965 until OBRA in 1981, state Medicaid programs had only limited control over hospital payments. States were required to use the Medicare principles of reimbursement on the basis of reasonable costs as the method to determine payments to hospitals for services to Medicaid beneficiaries.

The close link between Medicare and Medicaid policy for hospital payment resulted in Medicaid hospital payment levels comparable to those of Medicare and private insurers. As a result, hospitals did not face the kinds of reductions in payment levels under Medicaid that physicians had encountered since the early seventies, when states attempted to contain Medicaid costs by freezing physician payment levels or setting the levels well below private rates.

Prior to 1981, states had some authority to modify Medicaid hospital payment from the Medicare principles, but the authority was very limited. Under the 1972 Social Security Amendments, states could implement alternative methods for hospital payment under Medicaid, but such methods had to be based on reasonable costs (i.e., all costs incurred by the hospital for services provided to the Medicaid patient) and be approved by the Secretary of Health and Human Services. As shown in table 4.3, by 1980 eleven states had elected to pursue this approach, half of them rate-setting states (HCFA 1982; the state rate-setting programs are described in chapter 5).

With the passage of OBRA in 1981, Congress removed the requirement that a waiver was needed to decouple Medicaid hospital payment from Medicare reasonable-cost principles. States were given more flexibility to develop and implement new Medicaid hospital payment methods as long as those payments were reasonable and adequate to meet the costs of efficiently and economically operated facilities. The payment levels were to take into account the circumstances of hospitals serving a disproportionate number of low-income patients and be sufficient to ensure Medicaid patients reasonable access to services of adequate quality (Bovbjerg and Holahan 1982).

These conditions were intended to protect hospitals, especially public hospitals, serving large numbers of the poor by requiring states to give special consideration to such facilities in their payment methodologies. This provision means that states can set payment rates independent of the costs of any particular hospital and not related to increases in the

Table 4.3. **Medicaid Hospital Payment Methods, 1980 and 1986**

State	1980			1986		
	Medicare Methods	Methods Applying to Medicaid Only	Methods Applying to Medicaid and Other Payers	Medicare Method	Methods Applying to Medicaid Only	Methods Applying to Medicaid and Other Payers
Total Number	40	5	5	16	21	13
Alabama	X					X
Alaska	X				X	
Arizona[a]						
Arkansas	X				X	
California		X				X
Colorado		X			X	
Connecticut	X			X		
Delaware	X			X		
District of Columbia	X				X	
Florida	X				X	
Georgia	X				X	
Hawaii	X			X		
Idaho		X			X	
Illinois	X				X	
Indiana	X				X	
Iowa	X				X	
Kansas	X				X	
Kentucky	X			X		
Louisiana	X			X		
Maine	X					X
Maryland			X			X
Massachusetts			X			X
Michigan		X			X	
Minnesota	X			X		
Mississippi	X					X
Missouri	X				X	
Montana	X			X		
Nebraska	X					X
Nevada	X				X	
New Hampshire	X					X
New Jersey			X			X
New Mexico	X				X	
New York			X			X
North Carolina	X				X	
North Dakota	X			X		

Table 4.3. *Continued*

| | 1980 | | | 1986 | | |
| | Medicare Methods | Methods Applying to Medicaid Only | Methods Applying to Medicaid and Other Payers | Medicare Method | Methods Applying to Medicaid Only | Methods Applying to Medicaid and Other Payers |
State						
Ohio	X			X		
Oklahoma	X				X	
Oregon	X			X		
Pennsylvania		X		X		
Rhode Island			X			X
South Carolina	X			X		
South Dakota	X			X		
Tennessee	X					X
Texas	X			X		
Utah	X				X	
Vermont	X				X	
Virginia	X				X	
Washington	X				X	
West Virginia	X			X		
Wisconsin	X					X
Wyoming	X			X		

Sources: HCFA 1982, 1987a.

[a]Arizona had no program in these years.

costs of goods and services purchased by the hospitals. Prior to OBRA, HCFA would not have approved such alternate plans. In addition to modifying the conditions for approval, OBRA also streamlined the HCFA approval process for alternative plans to make state changes faster and easier to implement.

Implementation of the 1981 OBRA hospital payment provisions by the states was accelerated by the changes in Medicare hospital payment enacted in 1982 and 1983 described in chapter 3. In 1982 TEFRA set a ceiling on Medicare hospital payment levels, and in 1983 Congress enacted the Medicare Prospective Payment System using DRGs to replace payment on a cost basis. The Medicare hospital payment changes meant that many states could no longer rely on Medicare payment methodology and avoid revisions to their own Medicaid hospital payment system.

Most states moved to develop their own payment methodology, and others are in the process of changing. All the new plans were directed solely at Medicaid hospital payments and did not tie Medicaid to all-payer reforms, as most of the earlier alternative systems had done. As shown in table 4.3, by 1986 only sixteen states continued to use the Medicare principles of reasonable-cost reimbursement as their Medicaid payment policy (HCFA 1987b). Twenty-four states developed new plans between 1980 and 1986. Both California and Michigan, with alternative Medicaid plans approved prior to 1981, implemented new payment methodologies in January 1982 under the new OBRA authority (Bovbjerg and Holahan 1982).

The new system implemented in California in 1982 represents one of the most dramatic changes in hospital payment under Medicaid. California converted its hospital payment approach to selective contracting on the basis of price, with the payment for providing services negotiated. Since 1983 a nine-member board has negotiated with providers and excluded any hospital that did not meet the price criteria (Olinger 1986). Hospitals with teaching programs and a high volume of Medicaid patients were most likely to win contracts, but the negotiated rates tended to be below the previous year's rates. These lower rates resulted in the desired savings for the state (Brown, Cousineau, and Price 1985). A study of the early results in California found that the contracting system, combined with utilization controls, reduced Medicaid per diem rates by 19 percent and prevented any offsetting volume increases (Feder and Holahan 1985). The selective contracting process saved $184 million from 1983 to 1984 and is estimated to have saved an additional $235 million from 1984 to 1985 (Johns, Anderson, and Derzon 1985).

In general, the new payment plans implemented after the OBRA legislation appear to have slowed the growth of hospital expenditures in the short time since their implementation. One study shows that average annual growth in hospital expenditures in states with new payment methods dropped from 15.7 percent from 1979 to 1981 to 8.5 percent from 1981 to 1983 (Cromwell and Hurdle 1984). The states that implemented new systems did not restrain cost increases quite as well as the states that changed their hospital payment systems prior to OBRA legislation, but they held cost increases lower than did the states that continued to use Medicare methods of reimbursement.

Medicaid hospital policy changes appear to have been effective in reducing the growth in expenditures per beneficiary from 3.8 percent from 1978 to 1981 to 0.9 percent from 1981 to 1984 (Holahan 1987). When aged, blind, and disabled beneficiaries covered by both Medicare and Medicaid are excluded, real growth in hospital spending per beneficiary fell to zero during this period.

Differences appear to exist, however, in the relative effectiveness of reimbursement methods. Rate setting has achieved lower rates of growth in hospital expenditures, lower levels of cost per day and per admission, and a reduction in labor intensity over other methods (Cromwell and

Kanak 1982; Kidder and Sullivan 1982). States that use all-payer rate setting are able to force down hospital prices for all payers, so growth in expenditures may decline further in those states than in states relying solely on Medicaid hospital payment systems. The states with payment systems that apply only to Medicaid appear to have temporary savings that may not be sustained over time, whereas rate-setting states appear to hold their savings margin over time.

In sum, states have embarked on new and often untested approaches to hospital payment reform ranging from minor modifications in cost reimbursement to prospective payment on the basis of case mix. Given the recent nature of many of these changes, very little is known about the impact. However, the decoupling of the Medicaid payment levels from those of Medicare has the potential for creating differentials between the rates Medicaid pays for care of the poor and the payment rates for those who are on Medicare or privately insured. If Medicaid rates drop significantly below the market rate for hospital care, these payment methods could have deleterious effects on access to hospital services by the poor as well as cause serious financial problems for the providers who care for a high volume of poor patients.

A study by the AHA signals the importance of monitoring changes in access to hospital care among the Medicaid population. The study found that Medicaid admissions accounted for 60 percent of the 1.6 percent drop in hospital admissions for the entire nonelderly population from 1981 to 1982 (Martin, Dolkart, and Freko 1984). This is especially significant because Medicaid accounts for only 10.5 percent of the total hospital admissions for the population under age sixty-five.

Prepayment and Managed Care

As states have looked for new ways to restrain costs, restructuring the provision of care in a more cost-effective manner emerged as a potential solution to the difficult choices confronting most states. The Medicaid population's use of hospital emergency rooms for routine care and relatively high inpatient hospital admission rates and lengths of stay have led some states to explore various forms of managed care. In a managed care situation, the Medicaid beneficiary no longer has full freedom to choose his or her provider. Instead, a health care provider or organization arranges and coordinates all care.

Providing Medicaid beneficiaries with a physician or other provider who could provide continuity and coordination of care is viewed as a way of both improving quality of care and constraining costs. HMOs and other prepaid care systems, as well as "case management" systems, that link the Medicaid enrollee with a specific provider or set of providers are models of managed care. Medicaid programs argue that if effective, these systems of care could help to stretch limited state dollars for care of the poor.

Before 1981, individual Medicaid beneficiaries were assured freedom of choice in the selection of providers. This meant that a Medicaid beneficiary could receive services from any qualified provider and could not be restricted to a specified set of providers. As part of the increased flexibility given to the states in OBRA, Congress authorized the states to experiment with alternative methods of organizing and delivering care that included limiting care to a specified set of providers. OBRA permitted states to apply to HCFA for "freedom of choice" waivers. Such a waiver permitted states to limit the number and types of providers that a Medicaid beneficiary could select for care and to "lock in" the beneficiary to a single provider entity for a given period of time. This change permitted states to use case management and prepaid care systems for their Medicaid population.

The 1981 legislative changes also broadened the definition of an HMO as a Medicaid provider and relaxed the requirements on states to contract with HMOs for care of Medicaid patients. Prior to 1981 states were permitted to enroll Medicaid beneficiaries only in prepaid plans that had no more than 50 percent of their enrollees on Medicare or Medicaid and that were federally qualified HMOs or federally funded community health centers. Under the OBRA legislation, states were allowed to establish their own qualification standards for Medicaid HMOs, and these HMOs were permitted to have enrollments that were up to 75 percent Medicare and Medicaid (Neuschler 1985b).

Medicaid programs have begun to use their authority to waive freedom of choice in order to test various approaches to case management, capitation, and primary care networks. Managed care has been implemented for a limited population of 1.5 million in twenty-nine states and the District of Columbia (Anderson and Fox 1987). Wisconsin has mounted the largest enrollment effort for a Medicaid population, but as discussed in the next section, only preliminary evidence on effectiveness and access implications is available (Rowland and Lyons 1987).

Arizona has implemented a managed care system for the state's poor population called the Arizona Health Care Cost Containment System (AHCCCS). The AHCCCS project has been implemented on a demonstration basis as an alternative to a full-scale Medicaid program and, as such, is unique among the states. The system combines prepaid capitation, competitive bidding for provider contracts, strict eligibility determinations, nominal copayments, and freedom of choice restrictions into a single system. However, major changes since its inception make it difficult to draw conclusions about its impact on access and costs.

Managed care approaches offer promise if care can be delivered to the Medicaid population more cost effectively without compromising quality or access to care. Experiences to date have been mostly positive, but it is too early to report empirical results (Anderson and Fox 1987). But despite the obvious merits of capitated plans with coordinated services, putting providers at risk for care to the poor requires cautious implementation and monitoring to avoid underutilization of services, poor treatment, and denial of emergency services (Iglehart 1983a; Neuschler 1985b).

The Wisconsin HMO Preferred Enrollment Initiative

The movement toward prepaid capitated care systems for the Medicaid population is one of the most significant changes in Medicaid structure and operation to occur during the 1980s. In order to assess the implications of this delivery system reform on Medicaid beneficiaries and providers, a case study of the Wisconsin Medicaid program was undertaken (Rowland and Lyons 1987). Although other states implemented case management and prepayment systems, the Wisconsin program changes were the most significant in terms of extensiveness of reform and the percentage of Medicaid beneficiaries covered in the state.

Traditionally, Wisconsin has had one of the most generous Medicaid programs, with liberal eligibility standards, a comprehensive benefit package, and relatively unrestricted provider payment rates. Faced with a deficit in the state budget and rapidly escalating Medicaid costs, the Wisconsin legislature enacted a major restructuring of the Medicaid program in 1983. Under the reform strategy, care for Medicaid beneficiaries was to be converted from fee-for-service to prepaid managed care.

The 1983 state statute took full advantage of the federal legislative changes in OBRA that opened up new prepayment options for Medicaid. The state Department of Health and Social Services was directed to implement an HMO Preferred Provider Initiative for the Medicaid AFDC population. Several changes were also adopted at the state level to expand HMO coverage for the general population in Wisconsin as well as for the poor. Closed-panel HMOs were allowed to operate under state law without federal qualification, and the benefit structure for state employees was revised to provide an economic incentive for them to enroll in HMOs.

Under the Medicaid HMO Preferred Provider Initiative, AFDC Medicaid beneficiaries in Milwaukee and Dane (Madison area) counties were required to choose an HMO as their source of care. The fee-for-service option was effectively eliminated for all AFDC Medicaid beneficiaries in these two counties. In Milwaukee, with its large population base, this initiative resulted in the enrollment of 110,000 Medicaid beneficiaries in prepaid plans over a six-month period.

The Wisconsin Medicaid HMO Preferred Provider Initiative had been in operation less than two years at the time of Rowland and Lyons's case study in 1986 (Rowland and Lyons 1987). Rigorous analysis of the impact of the initiative on cost, access to care, quality, or health status of Medicaid beneficiaries was premature; however, the early insights of state and local managers, providers, health plans, and beneficiaries offered valuable lessons for other states and localities interested in pursuing a similar approach.

The Wisconsin initiative shows that the conversion of Medicaid beneficiaries from a fee-for-service system to a capitated prepayment approach requires real commitment and careful planning on the part of state and local officials and active participation and support on the part of the provider community. Physicians and hospitals in Wisconsin formed new associations in order to continue participating in the provision of services to the Medicaid population.

Enrollment of the Medicaid population in HMOs was limited to young and routine-care Medicaid beneficiaries—AFDC children and their parents. Wisconsin did not attempt to enroll the aged or disabled beneficiaries into HMOs because they generally have Medicare as well Medicaid coverage and are more difficult to capitate because of their declining health status. Even within the AFDC population, hard-to-manage patients were excluded from the HMO initiative. AFDC families including a mentally retarded child or a member with severe mental health or drug abuse problems were excluded from the initiative and continued to receive care reimbursed on a fee-for-service basis. Thus, the participants in the HMO initiative were those with the most routine and predictable health care needs and therefore the easiest group to capitate. Before capitation can be applied more broadly to the full Medicaid population, a more sophisticated capitation method that reflects the variations in health status among the aged and the disabled and takes into account the health expenses of special population groups must be developed.

The Wisconsin initiative also reveals that implementation of broad-scale reform is easier if the capitation rates are generous and competitive with private rates. Wisconsin's method for setting capitation levels was based on a flat reduction of the fee-for-service estimated expenditures. The state estimated what it would have spent and then reduced that amount by 7 percent when seeking bids from the HMOs. The plan received the same capitation amount for each person regardless of age, sex, or health status. The reimbursement level was therefore generous because it was based on prior fee-for-service expenditures, which were high owing to the comprehensive benefit package and relatively unrestricted payment policies. The flat rate per enrollee regardless of age also means that plans with a greater than average proportion of children fare better than those with a proportionately larger adult population.

Both the participating plans and the state agreed that the initial payment levels were comparable to the private HMO rates and made care of the Medicaid population on a capitation basis economically feasible and in some cases economically attractive. However, the generous capitation levels are not expected to last because the state Medicaid program continues to be pressed by the legislature to contain costs and help reduce state spending. In the future the state intends to set capitation rates for participating plans based on a percentage reduction in the HMO average cost per enrollee instead of setting rates based on fee for service spending. Provider participants noted that as the state ratchets the rates down, the plans and especially the participating physicians are likely to become less willing to treat the Medicaid population.

Another major issue involved in the capitation rate determination concerns what services are to be covered by the plan. Specifically, in addition to basic medical services, the state requires the plan to cover emergency services and mental health care. Emergency services have been a major problem area for the HMOs. The AFDC Medicaid population has traditionally sought care for both emergencies and more routine services in the hospital emergency room. Much of this care has been provided in the evening, after traditional physician offices are closed. The HMO plans are unwilling to pay the hospitals for care delivered to their enrollees that is not truly emergency care, yet the patients need education and counseling to change their current patterns of care.

One of the innovative solutions to the emergency care coverage problems facing the participating plans is the triage system developed at Mount Sinai hospital. The HMO plans had difficulty maintaining twenty-four-hour physician coverage for emergency care. The hospital was being denied payment for rendering nonemergency care after hours. Under the new system, the hospital is under contract to the HMO plans, and its emergency room physicians provide consultation and screening for emergency care. This is an example of the cooperative arrangements that can be developed as traditional and new providers struggle to adapt to the new environment.

The Wisconsin experience also shows that such systems can only be implemented with coordination and frequent readjustment of arrangements at the local level. The county and the state are continually working to improve the eligibility process, the handling of court-assigned cases, and the provision of mental health and retardation benefits. Similarly, the issues raised in the provision of ambulance versus paramedic care point out the need to recognize when existing networks and relationships are in jeopardy and need to be realigned.

Finally, the Wisconsin experience points out that these projects take time to develop and that comprehensive HMO systems are not developed quickly. Only one of the participating plans in Milwaukee is a federally qualified staff-model HMO. All the other plans are Independent Practice Associations (IPAs), which are paid a capitation rate for care of the Medicaid population but reimburse their participating physicians using a discounted fee-for-service model. Most have been set up exclusively for this project and serve a predominantly poor population. However, the Wisconsin experience also demonstrates that the market will respond to economic incentives, and providers will adapt their practice arrangements to retain their patient base.

One of the major issues facing these plans in the future is whether they can attract privately insured patients. Federal law requires that plans participating in Medicaid have a mix of public and private patients after an initial phase-in period. Unless the plans are able to achieve this mix, the HMO initiative will have to be redirected to only those plans with integrated payers and an adequate privately insured market.

In summary, the Wisconsin HMO preferred provider initiative appears to show that a state can transfer care for Medicaid children and their families from a fee-for-service arrangement to prepaid plans without major disruption in the health care system or services to beneficiaries in the short run. However, the long-run consequences of this action cannot yet be evaluated. The Wisconsin effort demonstrates that care of special population groups, access to emergency room services, provision of specialized services, and coordination among providers as well as the state and county are all difficult issues that must be addressed and readdressed throughout implementation.

It is too early in the Wisconsin initiative to know what the project has meant for Medicaid beneficiaries' access to care and health status or for health care providers' quality of care and fiscal viability. The potential for providing inadequate levels of care to beneficiaries cannot be underestimated in a system where the fee-for-services option has been essentially eliminated for most AFDC beneficiaries.

Many questions remain unanswered. Has the system really saved money? Have the health plans provided a valuable service or just taken dollars away from services in their middleman role? Have beneficiaries really adjusted to the new system, or is their perception that care is rendered as before? What happens when the state really starts to squeeze down on payment rates for the plans? The impact of the project on cost, quality, and access to care requires careful evaluation before its success or failure can be pronounced.

Policy Implications of Payment Reform for the Poor

The Medicaid program has changed since 1980 in the face of an upsurge in both government and private sector health cost containment activity and budgetary and legislative changes at the federal level. In combination with the 1981 recession, OBRA added pressure on the states to control spending by reducing the federal matching rate if target growth rates were exceeded. To assist in restraining costs, states were given additional flexibility over program design and new authority over hospital payment. In response, most states implemented cost containment policies to try to restrain Medicaid spending. The state responses have been neither uniform nor comprehensive. Most states have employed a variety of policy instruments to curb spending. Each state has essentially fashioned its own approach, although there are clearly common elements in the strategies employed.

The impact of these changes on the scope and configuration of the Medicaid program nationwide are not yet known. Some changes, such as the new hospital payment system in California, are extensive and will be closely monitored and independently evaluated. Other changes, such as the increase in prior authorization as a requirement for hospital admission, are more subtle but could still significantly influence the willingness and ability of providers to admit Medicaid patients. Over the long term, many of these policies could have an impact on access to care for the poor.

Additional studies to determine whether Medicaid patients receive their health care differently as a consequence of the cutbacks in benefits and provider payment are needed. Such cutbacks may lead to a shift in the source of care for many of the poor from physicians' offices to hospital outpatient departments and from private to public hospitals, but these patterns have not been documented (Vladeck 1981). Similarly, hospital admissions for the poor and near-poor through the emergency room may increase while scheduled elective care decreases. Empirical evidence to document these changes is still lacking.

Clearly, the results of the legislative changes to the Medicaid program since 1980 are mixed. There were cutbacks and changes in program scope as a result of the Reagan administration, but there has also been progress in maintaining coverage for the poor. The attempt to cap federal Medicaid expenditures was defeated, and the entitlement nature of the program was preserved, although federal expenditures were cut and states were given more leeway over their Medicaid programs. Even with increased flexibility most states have maintained basic services.

Recent legislation has signaled recognition in Congress of the essential nature of Medicaid coverage of the poor, including expansion of coverage for pregnant women and children, exemption of Medicaid from the automatic cuts resulting from the Gramm-Rudman legislation, and inclusion of the option to cover the elderly, the disabled, young children, and pregnant women to the poverty level. There remains a great need for continued monitoring of the program to ensure that access to services and the quality of those services are maintained.

Chapter 5

**The Experience of State
Rate-setting Agencies**

State governments led the way in the 1970s in developing innovative hospital prospective payment systems. Often with federal funding, states developed alternative approaches to containing health care costs through implementation of rate-setting programs that had the authority to approve or set hospital rates or budgets. There were several motives for adopting these programs, including rising hospital costs contributing to rapid increases in state Medicaid outlays, concerns by certain payers that they were paying a greater percentage of total costs, the desire to avoid federal regulation, and the challenge of developing a model program with potential national application. This chapter reviews the experience of state rate-setting agencies, including the historical development of programs and empirical evidence on their effectiveness in containing costs. The chapter concludes with highlights of the major lessons learned from this experience and a proposal for future continuation of support for state rate-setting programs.

Definition and Characteristics of Rate-setting Programs

The regulation of hospital charges or costs at the state level began in earnest in the early 1970s. In 1974 Dowling found that twenty-two separate systems were in existence (Dowling 1974). By the end of 1985, rate-setting programs were in operation in thirty-five states (Merritt 1986).

Definition

Generically, the concept of state-level regulation of hospital rates involves an external authority (usually the state or a state agency but occasionally a private entity such as Blue Cross) that monitors each hospital's rates or budgets. Three important dimensions can be used to classify state rate-setting programs: (1) whether the program is mandatory or voluntary;

(2) whether it is regulatory or advisory; and (3) the method for setting rates.

Mandatory programs are those established by state law, which gives them legal power to require hospitals to submit to review and/or to force hospitals to comply with their directives. Voluntary programs, on the other hand, pose no sanctions for the hospitals' noncompliance; participation (and compliance) is left to the discretion of the hospitals. Regulatory programs have the ability to set hospital rates or budgets. Advisory programs, even though participation may be mandated by law, usually serve only to disclose, review, or compel the negotiation of hospitals' rates or budgets.

Experience in other industries suggests that voluntary programs are much less likely than mandatory programs to have an influence on hospital behavior and an impact on cost inflation. In voluntary programs hospitals can simply choose not to comply or even participate. Similarly, advisory programs are also less likely to be successful, since they rely on public pressure, uncertain negotiations, or the possibility of incentive payments as a means to change hospital behavior. Data from the rate-setting programs suggest that these hypotheses are valid.

In 1980 there were twenty-seven programs operating at the state level. As table 5.1 indicates, fifteen of the state-level programs in 1980 were voluntary. Four others required mandatory disclosure of hospital charges or budgets but otherwise had an advisory role. Eight states were mandatory-regulatory programs.

The emphasis of the balance of this chapter is on the states that operate mandatory-regulatory programs. Empirical studies have shown that these states had the greatest impact on hospital costs specifically and the health care delivery system more generally (Biles, Schramm, and Atkinson 1980; Coelen and Sullivan 1981). Particular attention is given to the four states (Maryland, Massachusetts, New Jersey, and New York) that have obtained and operated Medicare and Medicaid waivers, which permit the state agency to supplant Medicare's principles of reimbursement with its own, thereby bringing all payers within the jurisdiction of the agency.

Characteristics

The state programs have a number of features that are likely to affect hospital behavior. The most important features are (1) the unit of payment regulated, (2) the definition of allowable costs, (3) the adjustments and exceptions made to rates, and (4) the number of payers covered. Features of lesser importance include the responsible agency, the frequency of review and adjustment processes, and the nature of enforcement mechanisms and the appeals processes.

Table 5.1. Rate Regulation Programs by State, 1980

Mandatory-Regulatory	Mandatory-Advisory	Voluntary-Regulatory	Voluntary-Advisory
Connecticut	Arizona	Arkansas	Pennsylvania[a]
Illinois	Minnesota	Delaware	Wyoming
Maryland	Oregon	Florida	
Massachusetts	Virginia	Indiana	
New Jersey		Kansas	
New York		Kentucky	
Washington		Michigan	
Wisconsin		Missouri[a]	
		Montana	
		New Hampshire	
		Ohio[a]	
		Rhode Island	
		Vermont	

Source: Schramm et al. 1987.

Note: The source classified Missouri as mandatory-regulatory, which is incorrect; Missouri has been reclassified here and in the empirical analysis in this chapter. Colorado had a mandatory-regulatory program during part of the 1970s and is considered to have had such a program in the regression analysis. Although it is listed as mandatory-regulatory in this table source, Illinois never implemented its program, and the analysis in this chapter attributes no program to that state. The classification in some cases is debatable, in particular for Indiana and Rhode Island. However, with the exceptions noted above, the original American Hospital Association classification has been followed.

[a]Only part of the state was covered by rate regulation: Missouri, Blue Cross of Kansas City Plan Area; Ohio, Blue Cross of Southwest Ohio Plan Area; Pennsylvania, Blue Cross of Western Pennsylvania Plan Area.

The Unit of Payment Regulated

Perhaps the most crucial component of a rate-setting system is the unit of payment that is regulated. Prospective methodologies recognize that hospitals should be paid for their outputs and not their inputs. Therefore, most rely on some output unit as the basis for payment. Table 5.2 shows the various incentives that are created, depending on the unit of payment.

Most early regulatory programs set rates either for individual services (such as the price for a CT scan, various lab tests, or x-rays) or on the basis of a day of hospital care (per diem). As expected, establishing prices for individual services encourages hospitals to produce CT scans and lab tests more efficiently. It is also intuitive that payment on this basis creates no incentives for a hospital to reduce the number of services provided per day. Indeed, this choice may actually induce hospitals to provide *more* services if the price allowed exceeds the marginal cost of providing the service. Analogously, per diem rates, while they may discourage increases in tests or intensive services, create the obvious incentive to increase the length of stay in the hospital.

Table 5.2. **Incentives Inherent in Various Bases of Payments**

Basis of Payment	Incentives				
	Reduce Cost/Unit	Reduce Ancillary/Day	Reduce Length of Stay	Eliminate Admissions	Promote Regional Planning
Charges	Yes	No	No	No	No
Per diem	Yes	Yes	No·	No	No
Case	Yes	Yes	Yes	No	No
Total hospital budget	Yes	Yes	Yes	Yes	No
Regional limit capitation	Yes	Yes	Yes	Yes	Yes

Not surprisingly, many early programs (i.e., in Maryland and New York) that initially used per diem or per-service rates were confronted with increases in length of stay or increased utilization of certain services as a result of the unit of payment that had been chosen. As a result, state programs changed their method of payment. By 1980 Maryland and New Jersey had modified their methodologies to pay on a per-admission basis and included volume adjustments designed to pay only the variable costs associated with increases in admissions. New York, while still paying hospitals on a per-day basis, calculated the per diem rate based on a total budget constraint and subjected hospitals to stringent utilization controls.

Determination of the Base Rate and Future Increases

Two decisions are important in determining the actual hospital rate allowed: first, the initial rate calculation at the beginning of the program; and second, the method of increasing this rate over time. Most states have established the initial rate, called the base rate, on the basis of a review of each hospital's cost for "reasonableness." The determination of reasonableness may be based on a comparison of costs among similar hospitals or upon a review of the hospital's own costs. States differ in the extent to which the rate is set to cover the "full financial requirements" of the hospital, including, for example, an allowance to cover the costs of care for patients who cannot pay and have no insurance, the direct and indirect costs of graduate medical education, capital-related operating costs, working capital costs, and allowable profit levels. Similarly, the standards for screening or comparing hospitals with one another for purposes of determining allowable costs also differ.

The second important decision concerns how the rate is changed over time. The objective is to establish an independent standard to calculate an acceptable rate of increase. To avoid rewarding hospitals whose costs rise rapidly over time, it is important that the allowable increase not be calculated based on individual hospital cost increases. That is, future rates should be set independent of the costs incurred by the institution subsequent to its base year. A second concern is that if rate increases are tied to wage increases experienced by the hospital industry, hospitals will have no incentive to become wise consumers. To avoid this, rate increases should be tied to changes in the overall economy.

Most early programs were beset with the problem of setting rates in subsequent years by using the preceding year's cost. Of the mandatory-regulatory states, Massachusetts, New Jersey, New York, and Washington were the first to recognize this flaw, and by 1982 they had adopted payment rates that were not based on the previous year's cost. In these states, once reasonable rates for a base year were established, an inflation rate could be applied to generate rates for succeeding years. Further scrutiny of costs is made only at the hospital's request for a rate appeal or during occasional rebasings.

Adjustments and Exceptions Made to Rates

Annual or periodic adjustments to rates are typically made to account for at least two types of costs deemed beyond a hospital's control. First, inflation in the prices of the inputs, such as labor and supplies purchased by hospitals, is allowed. Most states use a market basket index (see chapter 3), although components and weights vary considerably across states. Second, since the types of patients seen at the hospital affects costs, most systems find it necessary to adjust for changes in the case mix of a hospital. New Jersey's program, which is the prototype for the Medicare PPS, directly accounts for case mix by paying on the basis of DRGs. Maryland permits a variety of patient classification schemes to be used for adjusting rates, although the trend is toward DRGs. New York uses case mix data for purposes of classifying hospitals into specific groups that are then used to determine adjustments.

State programs try to avoid giving hospitals an incentive to increase the number of services provided by using a comprehensive unit of payment, such as a rate per hospitalized patient. However, even this method of payment gives hospitals an incentive to increase the number of patients admitted. To discourage increasing utilization, most systems pay only for the variable costs associated with any increase in the number of patients.

The Number of Payers Covered

Another important feature of state rate-setting programs is the range of patients to which established rates apply. Many states began their programs with rates applying only to patients covered under the Medicaid program, Blue Cross, and private health insurance plans. In recent years a few states have expanded their programs to include Medicare and privately insured patients as well. These systems are called "all-payer" systems.

All-Payer Systems

While mandatory-regulatory state rate-setting initiatives have existed since the early 1970s, the all-payer concept has evolved only recently. Maryland instituted the first all-payer system—receiving a waiver from Medicare principles in 1977. The other three states (New York, New Jersey, and Massachusetts) received waivers in the early 1980s.

In order to institute an all-payer program, the state must decide to pay all payers under the same rules and obtain from HCFA a waiver of Medicare reimbursement principles. Receipt and maintenance of a Medicare waiver by a state is conditioned on a number of criteria, which are defined in Section 402 of the Social Security Amendments of 1967, as amended by Section 222(b) of the Social Security Amendments of 1972. The performance criterion for waivers granted under these provisions was that the rate of increase in the state in Medicare inpatient hospital payments, in aggregate or per Medicare inpatient admission, could not exceed the national rate of inflation for such payments over any thirty-six-month period. The rule was amended slightly by the 1983 Social Security Amendments.

The Impetus for State Rate Setting

The factors impelling the creation of state rate setting, especially of the all-payer variety, are nearly as varied as the systems themselves. Some programs, such as New York's, were mainly the result of incessant cost increases in an already costly Medicaid program during a time of dwindling state funds and a severe budget crisis in the late 1960s. Others, such as the Massachusetts program, were influenced by dramatic increases in private hospitalization insurance premiums and increases in employer contributions for employee benefits. In New Jersey the growing payment differential between Blue Cross and commercial insurers and the rising concern over cost shifting played a role. In still others, such as Maryland's, the financial distress of the industry, especially in Baltimore's inner-city hospitals, contributed to passage of legislation. While the factors that in the past engendered or fostered all-payer rate setting varied, certain common motivations were shared by the proponents. All are still valid and applicable today.

Cost Shifting

Perhaps the major impetus for all-payer rate setting is the desire to prevent cost shifting among payers and restore payer equity. In past years

Medicare has forced other payers to cover a larger share of a hospital's costs. This resulted from its principles of reimbursement with respect to bad debt, charity care, depreciation expense, and other items (Ginsburg and Sloan 1984).

Further, as a result of its large market share, close ties with the hospital industry, or adoption of Medicare's reimbursement principles, Blue Cross often paid less than other private payers. In addition, many early rate-setting initiatives that did not regulate all third-party payers exacerbated the problem of payer differentials. In 1974, primarily to protect the state's Medicaid budget, the New Jersey Department of Health began to regulate hospital payments made by Medicaid and Blue Cross. Blue Cross was included because the state was responsible for approving premium levels and was under pressure to keep increases low. Within five years, by its own account, Blue Cross in New Jersey was paying 30 percent less than the commercial insurers for similar patients in similar hospitals. Because the other payers were heavily subsidizing Blue Cross and Medicaid, Blue Cross began to realize an enormous competitive advantage in selling insurance.

Equitable Distribution of Uncompensated Care and Improved Access

Part of the appeal of all-payer rate setting is that hospitals are not discouraged from providing certain services, such as uncompensated care and graduate medical education. Under varying methodologies, the prospective systems in the four states have served to apportion the costs of these services among all payers, which removes the disincentives that exist in a competitive environment for hospitals to provide such services. Consequently, in contrast to the situation in states without rate-setting programs, access of the uninsured and underinsured to hospital services is preserved, if not improved. A further consequence is that the financial condition of those hospitals that historically have provided disproportionate amounts of charity care is usually protected.

Federal Encouragement of State Rate Setting

As early as 1967, Congress authorized experimentation with alternative reimbursement methodologies in its search for strategies to control hospital costs. However, federal encouragement of state rate setting (in the form of funds for research and operations) did not begin in earnest until 1972, with the passage of Section 222(b) of the Social Security Amendments of 1972 (see chapter 2). Federal interest in rate setting reached its peak during the Carter administration. The Carter Hospital Cost Containment Act of 1977, which would have established a national all-payer system, stipulated that rate-setting states that were successful in controlling cost inflation would be exempt from its provisions.

During the Reagan administration, congressional legislation continued to support state-level options, although the interest of the executive branch had clearly waned. OBRA encouraged the development of state prospective methodologies for the Medicaid program and provided financial incentives to states with rate-setting programs. Similarly, TEFRA reemphasized support for state approaches by specifying the conditions under which a Medicare waiver would be granted. Finally, in 1983, with the passage of the Social Security Amendments (which implemented the DRG-based PPS for Medicare), Congress moved to establish a nondiscretionary, statutory right to a Medicare waiver if certain criteria are met.

The Impact of State Rate Setting

The effectiveness of state rate-setting programs has been the subject of numerous studies. These studies have focused primarily on the impact of the programs in reducing the rate of increase in hospital costs. More recently, studies have documented the savings to Medicare in states with waivers releasing them from Medicare payment principles. Some studies have investigated other effects, such as their impact on utilization of health care services and hospital financial viability. Questions have been raised about the impact of such programs on quality of care, but this aspect has not been rigorously investigated because of the difficulties associated with monitoring quality of care.

The Impact on Costs

Econometric studies have demonstrated conclusively that state rate-setting programs are successful in reducing the rate of increase in hospital costs, and the effectiveness of such programs in this regard is no longer seriously contested (Biles, Schramm, and Atkinson 1980; CBO 1979a; Schramm, Renn, and Biles 1986; Sloan, Feldman, and Steinwald 1983). Schramm, Renn, and Biles (1986) found that between 1976 and 1984 the rate of increase in hospital expenses per adjusted admission was 87 percent less in rate-setting states than in nonregulated states.

The results of the econometric studies provide little guidance as to which characteristics of rate-setting programs are likely to be important determinants of effectiveness. Coelen and Sullivan (1981) ranked, a priori, the nine programs they examined on the basis of relative program stringency. They concluded that their results were not consistent with the a priori rankings (for example, the Maryland program outperformed the cost containment predicted by its ranking, while the Washington program underperformed), and they were unable to find a common denominator that distinguished effective programs from ineffective ones.

Several tentative generalizations can be gleaned, however, from the experience of the mandatory-regulatory programs. First, Medicare participation is not a necessary condition for program effectiveness. For example, direct control over only a few minor payers (such as commercial insurers and self-payers in Connecticut) does not preclude program effectiveness. Second, the review and regulation of charges or costs at the hospital departmental level is not an essential feature of program efficacy. Nearly all of the states consistently found to be effective in lowering the rate of cost inflation (e.g., Maryland and Massachusetts) conduct reviews of only total budgets or aggregate spending levels for most of the regulated hospitals. Our conclusion is that rate setting is most effective in changing the style of medical practice and the aggregate production of hospital care and not the cost of an individual x-ray or lab test. In other words, rate-setting programs with a comprehensive unit of payment, such as a rate per admission, that provide an incentive to hospitals to reduce the number and intensity of services (such as length of stay, number of complex tests, etc.) appear to be more successful than those that regulate costs per service.

Other Effects

In addition to examining the effectiveness of state rate-setting programs in containing costs, some studies have investigated the spillover effects of state rate setting (e.g., its impact on the utilization of hospital services, the profitability of hospitals, the acquisition and use of capital by hospitals, the potential unbundling of services, and quality of care). As discussed above, the effect of rate setting on hospital utilization depends largely on the unit of output regulated. Early methodologies that set payment for units of service inadvertently encouraged the provision of more units of service per day, more days per case, and potentially more admissions per capita. At the opposite extreme, programs that establish global budgets (or set capitated rates) should induce hospitals to reduce intensity, decrease lengths of stay, and perhaps reduce the number of hospital admissions.

Most research to date has focused on the impact of rate setting on hospital expense per day, per admission, and per capita. Indirect inferences about rate setting's effect on hospital utilization can be derived by examining differences among the above outcome measures. For example, since expense per admission is the product of expense per day and length of stay, a difference between rate setting's effect on per-day and per-admission measures is due to a change in length of stay. Similarly, since per capita expense is the product of expense per admission and admissions per capita, differences between rate setting's effect on per-day and per-admission measures are due to changes in admission rates.

In the most comprehensive analysis of the effect of rate setting on hospital utilization, Worthington and Piro (1982) examined the nine ju-risdictions evaluated under the National Hospital Rate-setting Study from 1969 to 1978. They found that rate setting increased length of stay in states using the patient day as the payment unit but that few programs had a measurable effect on rates of hospital admissions.

Some studies have noted the deleterious effects of rate setting on the profitability of the regulated hospital industry (Hospital Association of New York State 1978; Mitchell 1982). Nearly all accounts stress the strin-gency of the New York program during the 1970s, which was unique. Most agree that as a group the hospitals in the mandatory rate-setting states have been consistently less profitable than those in states without programs. However, save for anecdotal evidence on the New York ex-perience, there is no empirical support for the claim that rate setting has impaired the access to or the acquisition of capital by hospitals. Further, recent studies indicate that, controlling for a number of pertinent factors, mandatory programs have had no effect on hospital profitability (Sloan 1981). Schramm, Renn, and Biles (1986) found that in the period 1976–84 operating margins of hospitals in regulated states improved and the difference in operating margins between regulated and unregulated states remained the same. Similarly, there is no evidence to date that rate setting has shifted care to outpatient or other ambulatory care settings.

Recent Trends

Federal legislative changes and, what is more important, the passage of the Medicare PPS legislation have made it difficult for all-payer rate-settings programs to continue. According to the PPS legislation, expen-ditures cannot exceed what Medicare would have paid absent a state reimbursement control system. As shown in chapter 3, these have been held to low levels of increase in recent years. This has meant that hospitals operating under state rate-setting programs have had all of their revenues held to the rates of increase in the Medicare program. This factor was the primary reason why New York and Massachusetts decided to drop Medicare from their all-payer systems. Hospitals also recognized that profit margins in the Medicare program were much higher than they were under the state programs, and they wanted to take advantage of the ability to earn profits.

Major Lessons

Since research frequently yields conflicting or ambiguous results, it is refreshing that in the case of state rate-setting the empirical results are clear and consistent: mandatory state rate-setting programs do significantly slow the rate of increase in hospital costs, with estimates indicating a rate about 3 percent slower in states with programs than in states without such programs. In 1984 hospital costs per adjusted admission in rate-setting states would have been 87 percent higher had these states not introduced programs (Schramm, Renn, and Biles 1986). State programs that have a comprehensive unit of payment, such as a rate per admission, have had better results. All-payer systems appear to work well, although mandatory state rate-setting programs without a Medicare waiver that cover only privately insured patients appear to have been effective as well.

State programs have achieved a number of objectives in addition to limiting the rise in hospital costs. They have contained provisions to pay for care of individuals without health insurance or with inadequate health insurance. They have assured contributions from all insurance plans for other nonpaying services, such as graduate medical education. They have achieved greater equity among payers by eliminating the differential between Blue Cross and commercial payers. They have prevented the deterioration in access to care for Medicaid patients that has occurred in states clamping down on hospital payment rates only for Medicaid patients. State prospective payment systems, such as the one in New Jersey, made a major contribution to the development of the Medicare PPS. They demonstrated that such systems are administratively workable and that they can be effective in changing hospital behavior and controlling costs.

Future Directions

Given the proven performance of state mandatory all-payer rate-setting programs in containing the rate of increase in hospital costs over a long period of time, every effort should be made to continue such systems where they exist and to permit additional states to enact such systems. The following recommendations are set forth to encourage effective state rate-setting systems:

• Federal cost containment provisions should be waived in states with mandatory, all-payer rate-setting systems meeting state-by-state targets on rate of increases in hospital expenses per capita.

• State programs must include provisions to ensure adequate care for the poor and the support of graduate medical education.

Chapter 6   **Corporate Cost Containment Initiatives**

Private sector initiatives to slow the rate of increase in health care costs have come primarily from major corporations concerned about rising employee health plan expenditures. Since thousands of companies have independently developed approaches to health care cost containment for their own workforce, interventions vary widely. Careful evaluations of different approaches are virtually nonexistent, but a body of evidence is accumulating to characterize the nature of changes adopted.

This chapter reviews the factors that led corporations in the early 1980s to pay greater attention to employee health benefits and to modify those benefit plans to foster greater economy. It also reviews the major types of changes adopted and the evidence available on the effectiveness of these changes. The emergence of preferred provider organizations, or PPOs, as a means to achieve lower-cost health care for employees is an important new phenomenon and is discussed in some detail. The chapter concludes with some recommendations regarding the future direction of employee health plans and their implications.

Trends in Employee Health Benefits

Employer payments for group health insurance have increased steadily over time. In 1950 employers paid less than $1 billion on group health insurance. By 1970 they were spending $12 billion. The period 1970–84 witnessed a sharp upward surge in group health insurance expenses: by 1984 employers were spending $93 billion, up 90 percent from the $49 billion spent just four years earlier, in 1980 (see fig. 6.1 and table 6.1).

Ninety-seven percent of all companies report insurance payments for health insurance coverage (Chamber of Commerce 1985). In 1984 health

Note: This chapter was written with the assistance of Steven C. Renn, J.D.

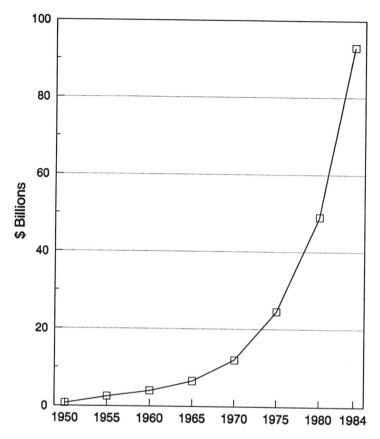

Fig. 6.1 **Employer Contributions to Group Health Insurance, 1950–1984**
(*Source:* U.S. Chamber of Commerce 1985, p. 31.)

insurance payments averaged 6.7 percent of payroll for manufacturing industries and 5.2 percent of payroll for nonmanufacturing industries, ranging from 3.5 percent for department stores to 8.9 percent for primary metal industries.

Group health insurance expenses are not the only health-related expenses employers incur. In 1984 employers paid a total of $2,385 per employee on health care costs broadly defined, or 11.1 percent of gross payroll. This included $1,391 per employee for group health insurance expenses, $262 for Medicare payroll taxes, $262 for workermen's compensation taxes, $111 for disability payments, $272 for paid sick leave, and $85 for dental insurance (see table 6.2). Employers clearly have a vested interest in a healthy workforce because of its implications for

Table 6.1. **Employer Contributions to Group Health Insurance, Selected Years, 1950–1984**

Year	Employer Contributions ($ billions)	Year	Employer Contributions ($ billions)
1950	$0.8	1975	24.0
1960	3.4	1980	48.9
1965	5.9	1984	92.6
1970	12.1		

Source: Chamber of Commerce, 1985, p. 31.

productivity, absenteeism, and health or health-related costs to the company.

A Climate for Change in Corporate Health Benefit Plans

Corporate action to institute cost containment provisions in employee health benefit plans did not begin in earnest until the 1980s. A survey of sixty-nine firms in 1980 (half of which were selected at random from *Fortune* lists and others from companies in Minneapolis, Rochester, and Boston) found that most of the firms had little impetus to seek changes in health benefits (Sapolsky et al. 1981). Health benefits were being expanded, not reduced. Firms were especially reluctant to require employees to absorb a greater share of their own health care costs. Employers feared that tighter claims control would disrupt employee relations. Employers were lukewarm toward health maintenance organizations because HMO savings were viewed as problematical and because employers

Table 6.2. **Employer Health and Health-Related Costs, 1984**

Employer Costs	Cost per Employee	Cost as Percentage of Gross Payroll
Group health insurance	$1,391	6.47
Medicare taxes	262	1.22
Workmen's compensation	262	1.22
Disability payments	111	0.52
Paid sick leave	272	1.26
Dental insurance	85	.39
Total[a]	$2,385	11.10

Source: Chamber of Commerce, 1985, p. i.

[a]Columns do not total exactly due to rounding.

did not want to force employees to select one type of health service delivery system over another. The most common cost-saving action by corporations was to self-insure, retaining insurance companies to administer benefits. Health promotion programs were adopted because employees liked them, not because employers were convinced that they would save money in the long term.

By early 1982 this passive attitude was beginning to change. Iglehart reported that "American industry, historically a slumbering giant when it came to influencing the delivery of health-care services that it purchased, is awakening to the need to become a more sophisticated buyer of such services" (Iglehart 1982a). He stressed one overriding reason for this shift in attitude: "soaring costs are crimping profit margins as never before."

The early 1980s brought great stress to American industry. Major leaps in oil prices in 1974 and 1979 created a major shock to industry and economies all over the world. Inflation soared, and the United States pursued an extremely restrictive monetary policy to bring inflation down. Interest rates soared, attracting foreign investment in U.S. securities and spurring the value of the dollar relative to foreign currencies to new heights. Unemployment increased significantly. The strong dollar brought competition from firms in other countries as Americans began to purchase imports at a record rate. The automotive industry was hit especially hard as high oil prices and the lowering yen and Deutsche mark made smaller, fuel-efficient Japanese and West German automobiles especially attractive. U.S. sales and profit margins dropped precipitously.

The health care sector, however, was experiencing quite a different trend. Health care expenditures were skyrocketing. With the removal of any threat of federal legislation to contain hospital costs, hospital costs shot up at an annual rate of 18–20 percent in 1980 and 1981. These skyrocketing costs were translated into major leaps in employee health benefit expenditures, and business felt the squeeze. The federal government acted in 1982 to restrain spending on hospital care under Medicare with passage of the Tax Equity and Fiscal Responsibility Act. The corporate community became concerned that limits on payments to hospitals under Medicare would result in even greater rates of increase in charges to privately insured patients as hospitals sought to maintain revenues.

These pressures culminated in a very dramatic turnaround in corporate attitudes toward employee benefit plans. Corporations demanded that employee benefit managers and private insurance companies administering their claims develop effective cost containment strategies. Health data analysis firms sprang up to respond to this new interest. Private foundations, government, and insurance companies all encouraged a more aggressive role for corporate America in dealing with the health care cost problem (Robert Wood Johnson Foundation 1982). Willingness to bargain toughly with unions to limit health benefits in an era when even wage giveback demands were part of the negotiation became a fact of corporate life. The expanding supply of physicians and the surplus of hospital beds further contributed to management's ability to take a more active role in negotiating attractive rates for employees.

The climate for a new era in employee benefit plans was thus altered by a host of factors emanating out of both the health sector and broader economic forces at play. While corporate interest was awakened, no obvious channel for this interest was apparent. Little hard evidence was available on effective cost containment approaches that employers could adopt independently without concerted action by all payers (Davis 1983). Experimentation with a wide variety of approaches became the order of the day. Rather than adopt any single strategy, many corporations adopted a multipronged approach including benefit redesign (largely greater use of deductible and copayment provisions), utilization and claims review, greater emphasis on employee enrollment in HMOs, and employee wellness programs (Fox, Goldbeck, and Spies 1984). Most recently, PPOs have been developed by insurance companies, provider groups, and entrepreneurs as a means of obtaining price discounts for employees who agree to obtain their care from a preferred list of physicians and/or hospitals (deLissovoy et al. 1986). In a very short period of time, cost containment measures previously believed to be unthinkable or unacceptable to both management and labor became standard practice.

Corporate Cost Containment Initiatives in the 1980s

Corporate cost containment initiatives in the 1980s took four major forms: greater employee sharing in the cost of health care services, direct measures to reduce utilization of health care services, encouragement of HMO or PPO enrollment by employees, and employee wellness programs. The most common of these was increased employee cost sharing. Most senior executives and corporate benefits officers believe that the changes they have instituted have helped curb health care costs (Louis Harris and Associates 1985). The trend toward self-insurance by large firms has continued in the 1980s, but since its impact is largely on the insurance industry rather than on health care providers, it is not dealt with in this book.

Cost Sharing

Employee sharing of health care expenses can take several forms. The employee can be required to pay a portion of the premium for health care benefits, either for his or her own coverage or for that of dependents.

Patient sharing in the direct cost of health care services use is referred to as cost sharing; this includes deductibles, coinsurance, or copayments. The deductible is the fixed amount that must be paid by the patient before insurance benefits begin. Coinsurance is the percentage contribution patients pay once the deductible is exceeded. Copayments are typically a fixed contribution (rather than a percentage contribution) toward each unit of service. A plan might, for example, require patients to pay a deductible of $150, 20 percent coinsurance on all hospital and physician expenses over $150, and a $1 copayment toward each prescription drug. Occasionally, the term "copayment" may be used more generically to refer to coinsurance (or a percentage contribution) as well as fixed payments per unit of service.

Cost sharing can reduce health care costs in two ways. First, it reduces the cost to the employer directly, as the employee is required to pick up expenses that would otherwise be paid by the employer. Employers, however, may compensate for the shifting in costs by expanding benefits (such as dental care or nonhealth benefits) or by raising wages more than they otherwise would have. Second, studies now demonstrate fairly conclusively that increased cost sharing in the form of deductibles or coinsurance reduces the total use of health care services (Newhouse et al. 1981). This is genuine expenditure reduction, but it may or may not reflect improved efficiency. One study has found little correspondence between the kind of reduced hospital utilization caused by patient cost sharing and unnecessary hospital utilization as judged by physicians (Siu et al. 1986). The health consequences of reduced utilization caused by higher cost sharing are still in some dispute. Several studies have found adverse health effects caused by cost sharing especially for low-income patients and patients with serious health problems (Brook et al. 1983; Hadley 1982; Lurie et al. 1984; Ware et al. 1986).

The appeal of increased cost sharing to employers in the early 1980s is not hard to understand. Companies were under tremendous pressure to reduce health benefit plan costs, and employee cost sharing was almost a guaranteed way to do so, both because of the potential for shifting costs to employees and because of the solid research results indicating that increased cost sharing reduces health care utilization. Employee contributions toward premiums can also reduce costs by inducing families with two or more workers to coordinate benefit coverage. For example, an employee may drop health coverage if already covered under a spouse's employer plan, or at least drop dependent coverage.

The major source of detailed, disaggregated data on employee health coverage is governmentally funded household interview surveys. Unfortunately, these surveys are expensive to mount and are conducted only about every ten years, and the data are reported with a considerable

Table 6.3. Cost-Sharing Health Plan Changes Made in the Three-Year Period 1982–1985

Change	Percentage of Companies
Changed to a contributory plan	21
Introduced deductible	24
Increased deductible	50
Introduced copayments	22
Increased copayments	27

Source: Louis Harris and Associates, 1985.

time lag. The latest available data from this source are for 1977 and are of no value in detecting trends in the early 1980s. Private companies have tried to fill this void with mail or telephone surveys of corporate executives or employees. These surveys suffer from unrepresentative samples, small sample sizes, low response rates, and emphasis on opinion questions rather than carefully cross-verified data.

Table 6.3 presents results from one of the best of the current surveys. It was sponsored by the Equitable Life Assurance Society of the United States and was conducted by Louis Harris and Associates. This survey covered a representative national cross section of 1,253 employees in corporations having five hundred or more employees, as well as interviews with a representative national cross section of senior executives, corporate benefit officers, and senior human resource executives in corporations having five hundred or more employees. Interviews were conducted in February and March 1985. As shown in table 6.3, many large firms have increased cost sharing in the last three years. Forty-five percent of all companies introduced or increased deductibles, and 49 percent of all companies introduced or increased copayments (or coinsurance provisions). About 50 percent of employees reported that cost sharing was increased somewhat or a great deal over the three-year period.

Other studies and surveys confirm the Equitable finding that employers have been increasing cost sharing. A survey by the A. H. Hansen Company of 861 firms of varying sizes in the fall of 1985 found that only 22 percent still provided health insurance benefits to their employees and dependents at no cost (A. S. Hansen, Inc. 1985). Thirty-three percent of the companies surveyed indicated that in the past two years they had increased employees' contributions to premiums; 43 percent indicated that they had increased deductibles; and 33 percent had increased their copayment requirements.

Hewitt Associates surveyed salaried employee benefit plans in 250 major U.S. companies annually from 1979 to 1984 (Hewitt Associates

1985). They found that the percentage of plans with a deductible for inpatient hospital services rose from 30 percent in 1982 to 63 percent in 1984. Similarly, the percentage of plans with a deductible for surgical charges rose from 34 percent in 1982 to 59 percent in 1984. Many firms increased deductible amounts over the period. In 1982, 82 percent of plans had a per-person deductible of $100 or less; in 1984 this percentage was down to 51 percent. The biggest movement has been to deductibles of $150–200 per year. Other changes reported by Hewitt include increased use of coinsurance and increased employee premium contributions. The percentage of companies requiring employee premium contributions for employee-only coverage increased from 31 percent in 1982 to 40 percent in 1984. Those requiring employee contributions for family coverage rose from 62 percent to 69 percent in the same period.

The Hewitt survey found, however, that reduced benefits in the form of higher cost sharing were frequently combined with improved benefits in the form of maximum ceilings on coinsurance payments by employees. A stop-loss provision, according to which the plan pays 100 percent of expenses once a certain level of employee outlay is reached, increased from 74 percent in 1982 to 87 percent in 1984. Higher lifetime maximum benefits have also been adopted. In 1979 only 13 percent of plans with lifetime maximums specified a maximum larger than $250,000, compared with 59 percent in 1984. Employers have also softened the financial impact of higher cost-sharing provisions by implementing medical and dental reimbursement accounts, thus permitting employees to make required contributions on a pre-tax basis. In 1984, 18 percent of companies had a pre-tax payment option (Hewitt Associates 1985).

Changes in benefit coverage for salaried employees are an important early indicator of changes in coverage for all workers, since many union contracts require that any reduction in benefits be tried first in salaried employee plans. The Equitable survey found that of firms with unionized employees, changes in health plans applied mainly to nonunion employees in half the firms, while in the other half union and nonunion employees were affected equally (Louis Harris and Associates 1985).

Fox, Goldbeck, and Spies (1984) found that companies instituting cost sharing followed many different approaches. The Jones and Laughlin Steel Company and the Xerox Corporation related cost sharing to employee wages. In January 1983, Jones and Laughlin required employees to pay a family annual deductible on nonhospital services of 1 percent of annualized wages. Expenses above the deductible are subject to 20 percent coinsurance, with a maximum out-of-pocket ceiling of 3 percent of wages. Xerox introduced a similar feature in its salaried worker coverage in January 1984. The Equitable survey, however, found that only 7 percent of all companies had introduced a salary-related deductible program in the 1982–85 period (Louis Harris and Associates 1985).

Another approach to encouraging employees to reduce health care utilization is the medical expense account (Fox, Goldbeck, and Spies 1984). A medical expense account is a separate account for each employee from which money can be drawn to pay out-of-pocket health expenses, including premiums, cost sharing, and noncovered benefits. Any money not used can be carried forward to a future year or returned to the employee in cash. Cash refunds are taxable, while firms do not consider the use of the medical expense account to pay medical expenses to be taxable income to the employee.

Effective in January 1983, the Quaker Company established a $300 medical expense account; at the same time it instituted a $300 deductible and 15 percent coinsurance health plan (Fox, Goldbeck, and Spies 1984). It estimated that if no change in health care utilization occurred, the cost to the employer would be the same; however, if the employee reduced health care utilization in order to avoid drawing on the medical expense account, the company would save money. Xerox instituted a medical expense account of $400 per employee in 1984 and estimated that savings from reduced utilization would be 5–10 percent of premiums (Fox, Goldbeck, and Spies 1984). Alcoa established a benefits bank account of $700 per employee when it modified its plan to include a $700 maximum out-of-pocket health expenses ceiling (Stein 1985).

Another approach is the "cafeteria" or flexible benefit plan. According to this approach, the employer establishes a fixed dollar contribution to a range of benefits, such as group health insurance, life insurance, and dependent care. Typically, several health plan options are included. Employees can use the employer dollar contribution to cover a comprehensive health plan with little cost sharing, a health plan with high deductibles and major medical coverage combined with better life insurance coverage, and so on. Flexible benefit plans have the following advantages:

• They permit employees to tailor benefit packages to their own preferences

• They permit families with two or more workers to coordinate rather than duplicate employer fringe benefits

• They make the employer contribution more visible.

One disadvantage to workers is that this approach permits employers to cap or limit their financial liability for a range of fringe benefits.

Flexible benefit plans can be difficult to administer, can lead to adverse risk selection, and can contribute to employee dissatisfaction if poor choices are made (Fox, Goldbeck, and Spies 1984; Herzlinger and Schwartz 1985). PepsiCo is one example of a firm that has aggressively

Table 6.4. Selected Health Plan Changes Made in the Three-Year Period 1982–1985

Change	Percentage of Companies
Introduced second opinions	54
Introduced preadmission review	28
Initiated utilization review	27
Introduced plans to discourage hospitalization	47

Source: Louis Harris and Associates 1985.

pursued flexible benefits. In 1984 PepsiCo realigned the premiums to employees to reflect the relative cost of its health plan options and urged employees to opt for the health plan with lower premiums and larger out-of-pocket costs. Fifty percent of its employees moved to lower coverage and cost plans (Herzlinger and Schwartz 1985).

Measures to Reduce Health Care Utilization

In addition to financial incentives to patients to reduce utilization of health care services, employers have also been adopting direct measures to curb utilization, especially of costly hospital services. Such measures include: requiring employees to get a second opinion for surgery, preadmission review of all nonemergency hospital admissions, review of claims for medical necessity, prospective limits on length of hospital stay by diagnosis, and coverage of certain procedures only on an outpatient basis or strong financial incentives to shift care to an outpatient setting.

Measures to reduce the use of hospital care under employee health benefit plans have taken many forms. One of the most common measures is encouraging employees to obtain a second opinion before making a decision to have surgery. As shown in table 6.4, the Equitable survey found that 54 percent of companies introduced provisions for second opinions for surgery over the three-year period 1982–85. Mandatory second opinion programs are relatively rare (Health Research Institute 1981). More typically, firms give employees a financial incentive to obtain a second opinion. For example, since January 1983, Owens-Illinois's practice has been to pay 100 percent reimbursement for thirteen procedures if a second opinion is obtained but only 80 percent of both the surgeon's fee and hospitalization if it is not (Fox, Goldbeck, and Spies 1984). The thirteen procedures were those for which earlier studies had shown high nonconfirmation rates in the second opinion. May D&F introduced a $200 copayment penalty for cases in which a second opinion is not obtained. Prudential reports that about 10–15 percent of its large group plans have a second opinion program, of which 20 percent are voluntary and 80 percent have some form of incentive feature.

A second measure to reduce hospital use is utilization review. Utilization review may be prospective, that is, physicians may be required to obtain approval in advance before hospitalizing a patient in a nonemergency situation or to advise the hospital upon admission that the insurance plan will only pay for a fixed number of days depending upon the patient's diagnosis; or it may be retrospective and thus may lead to disallowance of charges for services deemed to be medically unnecessary.

Evidence on the extent of utilization review is mixed. As shown in table 6.4, the Equitable survey found that 28 percent of companies adopted preadmission review provisions and 27 percent increased utilization review over the 1982–85 period. Deere and Company in Iowa put a major emphasis on private utilization review (performed under contract with the Iowa Foundation for Medical Care) (Tell, Falik, and Fox 1984). Within a relatively short period of time Blue Cross, commercial insurers, and self-insured employers followed the lead of Deere, with the result that more than 80 percent of the private health insurance market in Iowa came under contract for private utilization review.

The Chrysler Corporation undertook a massive effort to winnow out unnecessary health care utilization and abuse of its employee health care plan in the early 1980s (Califano 1986). The three-year contract signed with the United Automobile Workers in October 1985 saved an estimated $50 million. Among the features of the new contract were:

- Hospital prescreening
- Employee choice of Blue Cross/Blue Shield, a PPO, or HMO options
- Preferred providers for vision care, laboratory tests, and podiatry services
- Incentives to reduce unnecessary use of emergency rooms (Califano 1986)

A third strategy adopted by corporations to discourage use of hospitals is to create incentives to obtain care on an ambulatory basis. Employer plans increasingly cover surgery on an ambulatory basis, and a few plans have better coverage for ambulatory surgery than for inpatient surgery. Philadelphia Blue Cross introduced provisions requiring that five types of surgery be performed on an outpatient basis (Lerner and Salkever 1983). Blue Cross of Michigan pays 25 percent more for twenty-six specific procedures when they are performed on an outpatient basis (Fox, Goldbeck, and Spies 1984).

The Hewitt survey found that many employers offer financial incentives that encourage employees to receive care on an ambulatory basis (Hewitt Associates 1985). Thirty-nine percent of companies used incentives for outpatient surgery, 37 percent for outpatient preadmission testing, and 25 percent for avoiding nonemergency use of emergency rooms.

HMOs

Federal legislation enacted in 1974 required employers to offer employees a choice of HMOs when they were available in the community. Corporate interest in encouraging employees to exercise this option mounted in the early 1980s. While clearly on the rise, the availability of an HMO option is not as widespread as might be believed: in 1985 only 32 percent of all employees in large firms had the option of enrollment in an HMO (Louis Harris and Associates 1985).

Many HMOs do not market to smaller firms, so the availability of this option is undoubtedly reduced for such workers. Rural areas do not typically have HMOs. Nationwide only 8 percent of the U.S. population currently belong to HMOs. HMOs tend to be most popular in areas with a young, highly mobile population and a high level of health care costs and supply (Tell, Falik, and Fox 1984). The characteristics of HMOs, their enrollees, and their experience are covered in greater detail in chapter 7.

PPOs

Definition

A new phenomenon beginning to affect employer health plans is the growth of preferred provider organizations (PPOs). A PPO is a plan that either restricts beneficiaries to a list of providers, such as hospitals and physicians, or provides financial incentives for beneficiaries to obtain their care from the list of preferred providers. In principle, selection of providers is based on price, that is, the lowest-cost hospitals or physicians willing to give substantial fee discounts are sought (Gabel and Ermann 1985). Providers may also be selected on the basis of lower expected utilization (e.g., physicians who historically have admitted a lower percentage of patients to hospitals or discharged patients more quickly). In addition, preferred providers are typically required to submit to utilization reviews and to alter practice patterns that reflect excessive use of health services. Some types of PPOs may use primary care physicians as "gatekeepers," requiring that beneficiaries obtain all their specialty care only by referral from the primary care physician. In 1985 an estimated 6 million people were covered by PPOs, with 44 percent of enrollees living in California (Rice et al. 1985).

PPOs differ from traditional health insurance plans in two major ways: (1) the insurer takes an active role in negotiating payment rates or selecting providers on the basis of lower expected cost to beneficiaries; and (2) the providers are on notice that they must comply with aggressive utilization review procedures.

PPOs differ from HMOs in several important respects. First, providers

Table 6.5. Sponsorship of PPOs

Category	Number	Percentage
Physician-hospital	96	23
Physicians	66	16
Hospitals	59	14
Blue Cross and Blue Shield combined	43	10
Other insurance carrier	40	10
Investor	26	6
Third-party administrator	22	5
IPA/HMOs	14	3
Self-insured employer	10	2
Other	37	9
Total	413	100

Source: AMCRA 1986.

are paid on a fee-for-service basis, not a capitation rate. Therefore, PPO providers are not at financial risk for services provided, nor is there a strong financial incentive on the part of providers to reduce utilization. Second, while beneficiaries have a financial incentive to use preferred providers, they typically may use providers outside the PPO plan. In an HMO use outside the plan is not covered. Third, relationships among providers within a PPO may be tenuous. Unlike many types of HMOs, PPO providers do not typically practice in a common location or in group practice arrangements. Fourth, PPOs are not subject to federal qualification, as are HMOs; therefore, there is no independent check on the financial soundness or quality of care of the PPO plan.

PPOs are sponsored by a wide variety of organizations. The major sponsors are providers (hospitals, physicians, and joint ventures of hospitals and physicians), insurance companies, third-party administrators, and entrepreneurs who act as negotiators with providers and marketers to employer groups. As shown in table 6.5, half of all PPOs are sponsored by providers. Insurance companies, however, may prove to be the most common sponsors in the future (deLissovoy et al. 1986). Insurance company–sponsored PPOs had 40 percent of all PPO enrollees in 1985 (Rice et al. 1985). Commercial insurance companies tend to select preferred hospitals on the basis of lowest costs, and physicians on the basis of lowest prices or utilization profiles. Provider-sponsored plans are less selective and are less concerned with the preferred provider's relative cost and utilization performance.

Incentives for PPO Development and Growth

PPOs are a natural reaction of employers anxious to avoid cost shifting by hospitals. Encouraging employees to select lower-cost providers through enrollment in a preferred provider plan has considerable appeal. By establishing a list of hospitals charging lower rates and urging employees and their dependents to obtain their care from such hospitals, employers can resist efforts of hospitals to recoup lost revenues from Medicare, Medicaid, and uninsured patients by charging patients covered under private insurance plans more. The success of the Medicare program and some state programs, such as California's, in setting or negotiating favorable rates with hospitals clearly pinpointed this as one fruitful avenue for private action (Johns, Anderson, and Derzon 1985).

Business has slowly awakened to the need to take an active role in negotiating the prices that hospitals and physicians will be paid for the care of employees and dependents. As Robert Burnett, chief executive officer of the Meredith Corporation in Des Moines, Iowa, said in an interview, "A corporation must be prepared to use the clout that comes with paying the bill for medical services if it is going to effect change" (Iglehart 1984a). The Equitable survey found that 9 percent of large firms initiated a PPO option over the three-year period 1982–85 (Louis Harris and Associates 1985). While this is a relatively small percentage, there is a strong indication that PPO plans will develop relatively rapidly. The Hansen survey of 861 firms found that although only 12 percent of employers have PPO arrangements now, 37 percent of those who do not are considering them (A. S. Hansen, Inc. 1985). A survey of *Fortune* 500 companies found that 16 percent of companies offered PPOs in 1984, up from 6 percent in 1983; and 30 percent of all companies surveyed expected to offer employees a PPO option in 1985 (Gardner, Kyzr, and Sabatino 1985).

There is some indication that PPOs flourish best when one or more large companies dominate the market for health services in a given geographic area (Tell, Falik, and Fox 1984). Rohr Industries in San Diego, for example, has been a leading force behind PPO development in that area. In Denver the PPO movement was initiated by the Martin E. Segal Company, a benefits consulting firm. Community support for PPOs in Denver was reinforced by Taft-Hartley union trust funds, which negotiate for health care dollar contributions and in turn are anxious to use those limited funds to obtain as many health care benefits as possible. By 1984, 100,000 trust fund members and their dependents in the Denver area were eligible to use one of the area's six PPOs, which represent approximately a thousand physicians and six hospitals (Tell, Falik, and Fox 1984).

PPOs have several sources of appeal for providers. First, their competitive orientation is philosophically more attuned to many providers than are HMOs or governmental programs. Second, with the increasing numbers of physicians and low hospital occupancy rates, PPOs offer the possibility of maintaining or increasing patient volume. Both physicians and hospitals are increasingly worried about having enough patients. Third, PPOs permit physicians to continue fee-for-service payment, which is the payment of choice of many physicians. Finally, PPOs often promise faster claims payment, which may improve provider cash flow. Providers, in turn, make two major concessions: willingness to provide care at lower rates and participation in utilization review.

Employees and dependents are likely to find PPOs attractive if they face lower premiums and cost sharing in a PPO option, if they can still use their current physicians or hospitals in their community, and if they have some assurance that the list of preferred providers is selected on a quality basis as well as a cost basis. Since there has been little emphasis to date on trying to assess quality of care from preferred providers, any poor-quality experience may lead to a backlash by employees and dependents.

PPO Growth and Future Prospects

The major increase in PPOs began in 1983. Prior to that date only 30 operational PPOs existed in the United States. By June 1986, 364 operational PPOs were identified (AMCRA 1986). An estimated 10.3 million people were eligible to use PPOs in 1986, up from 1.2 million in 1984 (AMCRA 1986; Rice et al. 1985). Since enrollees in most PPOs may continue to use nonpreferred providers, these figures overstate the full-time equivalent users of preferred providers. PPO activity, which seems to be concentrated in urban areas, is not dispersed equally across the United States; five states—California, Colorado, Florida, Illinois, and Ohio—contain half of the PPOs. California has 25 percent of the PPOs and 62 percent of enrollees (AMCRA 1986). For-profit PPOs, comprising 60 percent of the total, predominate in most geographic areas.

At least four factors should facilitate PPO development. First, a strong business presence in controlling health care costs and in assuming the role and risk of a self-funded insurer is conducive to PPO growth. Business coalitions typically heighten employer interest in cost containment and awareness about cost variations among providers in a given geographic area. Employer plans with a strong emphasis on utilization review and with a substantial employee base are in a strong position to negotiate actively with area providers.

Second, prior HMO growth in a region probably paves the way for PPO development. HMOs raise awareness of providers and insurers to alternative delivery systems. They represent a threat to the "market share" or patient loads of existing providers. Many providers, therefore, may see PPOs as a workable compromise between joining a capitated HMO and continuing fee-for-service reimbursement under a traditional health insurance plan.

Third, PPOs have flourished best in areas with excess capacity in hospital beds or physicians. Competition among hospitals and physicians for patients may make an area ripe for PPO activity.

Finally, a young, mobile population may be more conducive to PPO growth. As with those who enroll in HMOs, younger and more recently settled individuals have fewer and less-established ties with physicians and hospitals and are thus more amenable to restrictions placed on their choice of providers.

Surveys have verified the importance of some of these factors (Rice et al. 1985). The most common factors leading to PPO formation cited in a survey of PPO executives were competition from hospitals, physicians, and insurers stimulated by excess capacity. Cost containment pressures from employers and larger purchasers, such as pension funds, were cited by commercial insurers sponsoring PPOs (66 percent) and Blue Cross/Blue Shield plans (50 percent). Competition from HMOs was cited by 40 percent of hospital- and physician-sponsored plans and by 30 percent of Blue Cross/Blue Shield plans (Rice et al. 1985).

Regulation of PPOs

PPOs are a relatively new phenomenon and for the most part are not governed by specific statutes setting standards for performance. There is no federal qualification process to assure financial soundness or quality of care as there is with HMOs. Federal antitrust legislation and state-level legislation, however, have some effect on PPO operations.

Antitrust laws. In principle the emphasis on price competition by PPOs is consistent with antitrust laws. Several advisory business review letters by the Federal Trade Commission and the Department of Justice have offered favorable opinions of the PPO's procompetitive potential (Federal Trade Commission 1983; Department of Justice 1984). However, concerted action or agreements among providers relating to price (such as setting of uniform fee schedules or the amount of discounts from charges) or involving the exclusion of nonpreferred providers may be considered to be unreasonable or per se restraints of trade. Concerns may also be raised if a PPO plan has a large share of the market or a high proportion of area providers. In October 1984 the Stanislaus PPO of Modesto, California, disbanded under the threat of antitrust action by the U.S. Justice Department ("PPOs Face Antitrust Problems" 1984). The Stanislaus PPO had enrolled 50 percent of the doctors in Modesto and 90 percent of those in

Turlock on an exclusive basis, with a contract expressly prohibiting doctors from contracting with other PPOs or HMOs.

State regulation. If PPOs are sponsored by insurance companies or assume financial risk, typically they are subject to state insurance laws requiring the maintenance of adequate financial reserves, setting the form and content of provider and beneficiary agreements, and governing permissible types of investments. Some states have passed legislation governing PPO formation. Connecticut, for example, places specific limits on PPO discounts. Other states, such as Oregon, Oklahoma, and Virginia, have laws against discrimination in pricing of services, while still others make it illegal to sell services below costs ("PPOs Face Antitrust Problems" 1984).

Employee Wellness Programs

Larger employers have increasingly adopted employee health promotion or wellness programs. In 1985, 29 percent of employees in larger firms reported that their firm had such a program (Louis Harris and Associates 1985). In addition, 25 percent of employees reported that their firms had financial incentives to encourage employees to practice health and safety procedures such as not smoking, using seatbelts, exercising, or maintaining proper weight.

Worksite wellness programs take many forms. Programs include health risk appraisal that identifies diseases and biological risks that can lead to disease; behavioral change programs such as exercise programs, smoke-enders, weight loss programs, and stress management programs; health and safety measures in the workplace to reduce injuries and exposure to hazardous or toxic substances; and educational efforts (Fox, Goldbeck, and Spies 1984).

Corporations encourage employees to participate in wellness activities in a number of ways. Some try to heighten employee awareness by making mass screening and health risk appraisal tests and educational materials available at the worksite. Others make health enhancement programs and behavioral change programs (smoke-enders, weight loss programs, etc.) available at the worksite, for example by providing exercise facilities. Some companies give employees financial incentives to exercise, give up smoking, or lose weight. Hospital Corporation of America, for example, whose chief executive officer is a marathon runner, pays employees to engage in aerobic activities. Corporate culture can also be used to communicate the attitude that healthy habits are expected. PepsiCo, for example, promotes its products as having a young, healthy, vigorous image and similarly expects its employees to "Catch that Pepsi Spirit" (Fox, Goldbeck, and Spies 1984).

Two companies have developed extensive wellness programs for their employees, both because their company philosophies emphasize treating employees well and because they view the program as a marketable product. Johnson and Johnson developed the Live for Life program, which conducts annual health screens, makes health enhancement programs available at the worksite, and imbues healthy habits as part of the corporate culture. Control Data developed the STAYWELL program, which includes a confidential health risk profile and comprehensive sessions on behavior modification (Fox, Goldbeck, and Spies 1984).

The Effectiveness and Acceptability of Corporate Cost Containment Initiatives

Careful evaluations of the effectiveness of corporate cost containment initiatives are few in number. Since the multipronged corporate approach to cost containment has come at the same time as governmental changes and spontaneous changes in the health care marketplace, it is unlikely that the independent contribution of corporate cost containment measures can be assessed. Nonetheless, corporate officials widely believe that the measures instituted have been effective.

In firms instituting significant changes, over 90 percent of corporate benefits officers, senior executives, human resource executives, and brokers and consultants believe that the changes have been effective or somewhat effective (Louis Harris and Associates 1985). When these officials were asked to estimate in percentage terms how much higher health costs per employee would have been if the companies had not made changes over the three-year period 1982–85, the mean savings estimated was 17 percent. Interestingly, the estimated mean savings for different types of officials were quite similar: corporate benefits officers gave an estimate of 17.2 percent; senior executives, 16.3 percent; human resource executives, 17.9 percent; and brokers and consultants, 15.4 percent (Louis Harris and Associates 1985).

The Hewitt survey confirms many of these findings (Hewitt Associates 1985). Just under half of the companies covered by the survey (43 percent) felt that their cost management efforts had had a significant or moderate impact. Others felt either that the changes had had little impact or that they had not had sufficient time or data analysis to determine the actual effects. The Hewitt survey noted that the rate of increase in the cost of average medical claims per covered employee was expected to be 9 percent in 1984, down from the 15 percent increase experienced from 1982 to 1983.

Table 6.6. Acceptability and Effectiveness of Health Plan Changes Made in the
Three-Year Period 1982–1985

Change	Acceptability to Employees Affected (%)	Effectiveness as Perceived by Corporate Benefits Officers (%)
Changed to a contributory plan	68	71
Introduced deductibles	59	82
Increased deductibles	54	82
Introduced copayments	52	81
Increased copayments	48	78
Introduced plans to discourage hospitalization	83	81
Introduced preadmission review	73	73
Introduced second opinions	84	73
Initiated utilization reviews		67
Offered HMO option	80	49
Initiated a PPO	82	51
Started a wellness program	97	67
Instituted incentives for health and safety procedures	98	58
Started a health advisory service	98	49
Started a medical case management program	95	46
Offered a choice of two or more health plans	92	48
Introduced a disability case management program	96	52
Introduced a salary-related deductible program	80	39

Note: Acceptability is defined as the percentage of employees whose employers have made these changes who say that this kind of change is "very acceptable." Effectiveness is defined as the percentage of corporate benefits officers who say that this kind of change is "very effective" or "somewhat effective."
Source: Louis Harris and Associates 1985.

Cost Sharing

Among the corporate cost containment measures perceived by corporate officials to be very effective or somewhat effective, increased employee cost sharing rated highest (see table 6.6). Eighty percent of corporate benefits officers rated the introduction of or increase in deductibles and coinsurance as effective or somewhat effective in containing costs. The Hansen survey also found that employers believed employee cost sharing to be the most effective measure for containing costs; it was mentioned 60 percent more often than any other measure (A. S. Hansen, Inc. 1985).

A survey of all *Fortune* 500 companies and 250 industrials, of which 320 responded, found cost sharing the preferred option for cost containment, primarily because of its ease of implementation and relative effectiveness (Herzlinger and Schwartz 1985).

Many employees apparently grudgingly accept higher cost sharing. The Equitable survey found that half of employees in firms that made these changes said the changes were acceptable (Louis Harris and Associates 1985). Employers attempted to increase acceptability to employees by coupling increased cost sharing with expansion of other benefits, such as dental care or expanded outpatient benefits, and by mounting educational programs explaining the reasons for the changes in benefits. Unions, however, have voiced strong opposition to greater patient cost sharing. In 1983 the Communications Workers of America struck AT&T in part because of a proposal to increase employee health insurance premiums. Only after a joint labor-management committee reviewed a wide range of cost containment options were major changes agreed to (Abramowitz 1986).

Owen Bieber, president of the UAW, has recently expressed the all-out opposition of that major union to increased patient cost sharing: "Proposals to make consumers more cost conscious by shifting costs to them in the form of increased deductibles and copayments miss the mark. The UAW's opposition to increased patient cost sharing is not merely a reflex response to protect members' pocketbooks. The union resists, and will continue to resist, such mindless cost shifting, because it will not work. It does not get at the heart of the problem: provider driven overutilization and inflationary provider reimbursement systems. . . . The principal effect of cost sharing is to transfer the cost of services directly to the patient from the carrier or employer. It does not control costs, only shifts them" (Bieber 1985).

Union officials have expressed concern about the possible adverse effect on patients of patient cost sharing even when it is coupled with medical expense accounts to offset the financial effect. For example, Stein noted that the medical expense account idea is generally popular with employees but may do little for older, sicker workers. She quotes Cathy Schoen, of the Services Employees International Union: "The point in your career when you're the sickest is not the point you want your income to go down" (Stein 1985).

Measures to Reduce Hospitalization

Direct measures to reduce hospital utilization also receive high marks for their effectiveness and are considerably more acceptable to employees than is greater patient cost sharing. Preadmission review and second opinions for surgery were rated by 73 percent of corporate benefits officers in the Equitable survey as effective or somewhat effective (see table 6.6). A study of *Fortune* 500 companies that had executives rank the importance of health care cost containment strategies from 1 (lowest) to 10 (highest) gave high marks to a number of direct measures to encourage employees to obtain care outside the hospital setting: ambulatory surgery (8.3), outpatient testing (8.1), utilization review programs (7.7), second opinions for surgery (7.3), home care (7.3), preadmission review (7.1), concurrent review (6.7) (Gardner, Kyzr, and Sabatino 1985). Opinion surveys show much greater employee acceptance of measures to reduce hospital utilization than of cost sharing (see table 6.6). About 70–80 percent of employees found direct measures very acceptable.

Aside from these opinion surveys, careful evaluations are relatively rare. One innovation that has received careful scrutiny is second opinions for surgery. One study in New York found that 16 percent of individuals required by their insurance carriers to obtain a second opinion received a nonconfirmation of their surgery and that the benefit-cost ratio of this program was 2.6 (Ruchlin, Finkel, and McCarthy 1982). Another study of the mandatory second-opinion provision in the Massachusetts Medicaid program found that nonconfirmation rates averaged 14.5 percent, with a benefit-cost ratio between 3 and 4 (Martin et al. 1982). Brook and Lohr (1982), however, caution that "saving money is not the only issue— improving the quality of surgical care, protecting the ultimate health status of persons recommended for surgery, and ensuring social equity are equally important in the long run."

HMOs and PPOs

Offering an HMO or instituting a PPO was rated as effective by about half of corporate benefits officers in the Equitable survey (see table 6.6). Employers continue to have a "wait and see" attitude toward these approaches to containing costs, but they seem increasingly willing to offer them to employees. About 80 percent of employees find having these choices available very acceptable.

Wellness Programs

Two-thirds of corporate benefits officers surveyed by Equitable believed that starting a wellness program was effective in containing plan costs (see table 6.6). Wellness programs are extremely popular with employees; over 90 percent found them very acceptable. Careful evaluations of corporate wellness programs again are rare. The Johnson and Johnson Live for Life program has been evaluated using as controls employees in matched plant sites not offering the program. Evaluations have found reduced sick days, decreased smoking, and lower hospitalization costs for employees covered by the Live for Life program (Fox, Goldbeck, and

Spies 1984). Evaluation of the Control Data STAYWELL program has also found a significant effect on smoking cessation (Fox, Goldbeck, and Spies 1984).

Lessons from the Corporate Cost Containment Experience

The rapid rise in health care costs in the early 1980s hit the American corporate sector hard. It came at a time of deep recession and increasing competition from foreign markets. Federal health policy was focused almost exclusively on cost containment health care services provided to Medicare and Medicaid beneficiaries. These forces resulted in an unprecedented massive experiment in changing employee health benefit plans to foster greater efficiency and lower costs for employers.

Corporate cost containment initiatives have taken four major forms:

- Increased patient cost sharing
- Measures to reduce utilization of health care services, especially hospital care
- Encouraging employees to enroll in HMOs and PPOs
- Employee wellness programs

Careful evaluation of these initiatives is a long way off. Their independent contribution should prove difficult to establish; however, some general conclusions and caveats about corporate cost containment experience are possible.

Increased patient cost sharing and direct measures to reduce use of costly hospital services have been the favored strategies of corporations in the early 1980s. They are widely viewed by corporations as effective in slowing the rate of increase in premiums for employee health benefits and have encouraged employees to be more cost-conscious in the use of health care services. Reductions in hospitalization of the nonelderly in the early 1980s may be attributable to some degree to increased employee cost sharing and direct measures to curb hospital utilization (see chapter 3). Employers feel that these strategies have been reasonably acceptable to workers when accompanied by an educational campaign to explain the reasons for the changes.

There is a genuine question, however, whether increased cost sharing is in the best interest of workers. First, a lot of savings from the employers' perspective simply reflect a shifting of costs onto employees. As employees bear a larger share of the financial burden directly, it is likely that they will receive less health care. But this is not the same as improved efficiency, and it may have serious health consequences. Recent studies have shown that lower-income families and high-risk individuals can

Table 6.7. Employer Contributions to Group Health Insurance, Adjusted for Inflation

Year	Employer Payments (constant 1967 $ billions)
1950	1.1
1955	2.1
1960	3.8
1965	6.2
1970	10.4
1975	14.9
1980	19.8
1984	29.7
Annualized rate of change (%)	
1950–70	11.9
1970–80	6.7
1980–84	10.7

Source: Chamber of Commerce 1985.

suffer serious adverse health consequences when financial barriers deter them from seeking health care (Brook et al. 1983; Hadley 1982; Lurie et al. 1984).

Second, some of the savings are illusory. Inflation in the overall economy is down, and this dampening effect has worked its way slowly through the health sector. Real employer health insurance premiums rose 10.7 percent annually during the 1980–84 period, compared with 6.7 percent over the 1970–80 period (see table 6.7). It remains to be seen whether any real slowdown in employer premiums other than that attributed to a general improvement in inflation in the economy is occurring.

Third, many of the savings being achieved are likely to be one-time savings. That is, higher cost sharing and utilization review may shift costs down, but continued improvements are unlikely. For example, hospital stays can be shortened or certain procedures can be performed on an outpatient basis, but after a point no further reduction in hospital stay is achievable or humane, and certain conditions do require hospitalization. The longer-term prospect, therefore, is that the underlying rate of increase may well resume unless there are more fundamental shifts in the productive efficiency of the health system (Davis et al. 1985).

Another major lesson from corporate cost containment initiatives in the early 1980s is the emerging importance of PPOs. PPOs offer employers a way to identify lower-cost hospitals and physicians willing to charge lower prices and to encourage employees and dependents to obtain care from such a preferred set of providers. PPO enrollment seems likely to expand rapidly in future years. This development should be followed carefully to see whether PPOs prove to be effective in lowering total expenditures while providing quality care.

While PPOs provide employers with greater market power in the purchase of health care services, it should be remembered that other strategies could be even more effective. If all employers and public programs were to negotiate provider payment rates jointly, they would have even greater clout in the marketplace. A third-party bargaining unit should be able to dampen rates of increase over time much more successfully than one firm acting on behalf of even a large group of employees, since over time that firm would have to go along with increases that kept its employees attractive as patients relative to other patients.

From the point of view of social policy, three major concerns are raised by the growth of PPOs. First, growth of PPOs may further limit charity care and access to care for the uninsured. Hospitals cannot risk losing PPO business by trying to pass bad debts on to PPO patients. Second, preoccupation with cost may lead to too little attention to quality differences among providers. Lower-cost hospitals may be poor-quality institutions, and employees who have been encouraged or required to use such hospitals may be justifiably dismayed. Finally, favorable treatment of lower-cost hospitals may cause serious financial difficulties for teaching hospitals and further undermine support for graduate medical education and biomedical research.

Corporate interest in cost containment measures is a relatively recent phenomenon. As recently as 1980, employers expressed great hesitation about instituting any measures to curb the cost of employee health benefit plans. Will employer interest in these measures continue? The answer to this question depends upon several factors. Corporate health care cost containment initiatives are linked to general economic conditions facing firms. American industry has pulled out of the serious recession of the early 1980s, but economic growth and productivity are still weak, and competition from abroad is still a major problem. The sliding U.S. dollar should eventually reduce imports of foreign products and reduce some of the pressure on American industry, but economic pressures to keep labor costs down are likely to persist.

On the other hand, the drop in birth rates in the United States beginning in the mid-1960s means that fewer young people will be entering the labor market in the years ahead. Unemployment should decline, and firms should be under greater pressure to compete for workers. Good health benefits, especially for young families, are one of the attractions that firms can offer. Many corporations are genuinely concerned about the welfare of their workers and view it as good management practice to foster an image of caring and concern toward workers. Cost containment measures that are unacceptable to employees, such as greater and greater cost sharing or tough measures to restrict employees' freedom to choose their own health care provider, are unlikely to be adopted by such firms.

Trends in the health sector will also affect the degree of ongoing corporate interest and involvement. If corporations believe that health care costs are increasing at a relatively slower rate and that the health care cost problem has been solved, corporate interest should decline. A resurgence in increases in costs, however, could rekindle interest.

Evolution of the federal tax policy should also have implications for continued corporate cost containment initiatives. Loopholes in the tax code are permitting employees to pay many benefits with pretax dollars. If employees are able to pay health expenses out of pretax income or through medical expense accounts, then the distinction between health expenses paid by employers and expenses paid by employees begins to blur. Employers may increasingly decide to provide a fixed sum of money for health and other fringe benefits and give employees greater freedom to design their own mix of benefits. This approach helps corporations limit their financial liability, and it may be attractive to employees who have differing preferences regarding comprehensive health insurance, life insurance, day care, and other fringe benefits. While cafeteria plans allow employees to select less costly plans, they may also reduce the incentives of corporate benefits officers to adopt aggressive cost containment measures such as direct measures to limit the use of hospital care.

Most of these factors suggest a less aggressive role for corporations in the health care arena in future years. However, expanded choices for employees among plans with varying degrees of cost sharing, HMOs, and PPOs seem likely. Careful monitoring of the evolution of employee benefit plans and evaluation of the impact of these changes should provide important insight into the success of corporate cost containment initiatives over the longer term.

Future Policy Directions for Corporate Employee Health Plans

Corporate cost containment initiatives in the 1980s have been launched without major federal legislation and with very little outside assistance. For the most part it appears that this period of experimentation has been helpful. A wide variety of measures have been tried, without apparent harmful effects on workers and their dependents. There appear to have been some short-term savings—at least to employers and possibly to total health spending. Physicians, hospitals, and other health care providers have been placed on notice that their actions are subject to scrutiny by those who pay the bill, and the cost-consciousness of consumers has been raised. The long-term potential of current corporate cost containment initiatives, however, seems limited. Increases in patient cost sharing can achieve one-time savings, but continued increases in patient deductibles or coinsurance could cause lower-wage workers not to obtain necessary care and could lead to substantial employee and union dissatisfaction. Direct measures to curb hospital use are again one-time actions and unlikely to affect the rate of increase in health care premiums over time. HMO membership should continue to grow, but financial failures of some HMOs seem likely and will increase employer and employee wariness about these as a panacea for health care costs. PPOs have great potential, but their cost savings performance has yet to be demonstrated. Employers are likely to continue employee wellness programs, which should contribute to a general improvement in health awareness and habits.

National health policy could be directed toward encouraging employers to provide adequate health insurance coverage for all workers and to provide employers with more purchasing power. Specifically, federal legislation could mandate that all employers provide full-time employees with health insurance coverage meeting minimum standards and that hospitals, physicians, and other health care providers participating in Medicare be required to charge the same or lower rates to privately insured individuals enrolled in federally qualified preferred provider plans.

Congress has recently enacted legislation mandating that businesses with twenty or more employees that have employee health insurance plans must broaden the coverage of workers and dependents following termination of employment. Since July 1986, workers in firms having at least twenty employees must be covered for eighteen months following termination of employment, and widows, divorced spouses, and dependents must be covered for three years following death of the worker or divorce. Premiums must be equal to the employer group rate, but the individual, and not the employer, is required to pay the full premium. In addition, the beneficiaries must pay an additional 2 percent charge to cover administrative costs.

This recent expansion of coverage is an important step but falls short of the action needed. The major step needed is a requirement that employers provide at least some minimal health insurance to their workers. For example, Senator Edward M. Kennedy (D-Mass.) and others have proposed the employment minimum health benefits bill, which would require employers to provide coverage for all workers working at least $17\frac{1}{2}$ hours per week and their dependents.

The policy option proposed goes considerably further than recent changes. The first part of this policy option would mandate coverage of all full-time workers and their dependents under employer health plans and would establish minimum standards on the adequacy of coverage. Further details of such a proposal are outlined in chapter 12.

Chapter 7

Health Maintenance Organizations

It was not until the early 1970s, when federal interest in developing lower-cost health care alternatives increased sharply, that the concept of prepaid medical care really took hold in the United States. Today the health maintenance organization exemplifies this concept. Based on the experience of HMOs over the past two decades, many observers believe that HMOs constitute a promising vehicle for containing health care costs in the future.

The purpose of this chapter is to examine this premise by reviewing the growth of HMOs over the past two decades, examining recent trends in the HMO market, assessing the data pertaining to the cost-saving effects of HMOs, and considering the role HMOs are likely to play in the U.S. health care system in the future. The chapter is divided into seven sections. The first section describes the various types of HMOs that have come into existence. The second section reviews the federal policies that were implemented to encourage HMO development, the growth in HMOs that ensued, recent trends in the HMO market, and the demographic characteristics of HMO enrollees and disenrollees. The third section examines data pertaining to the extent to which HMOs provide care at less cost than the fee-for-service (FFS) sector does. The fourth section— based in part on a case study of HMO development in Baltimore which provides insight into policy issues related to HMOs and the role HMOs are likely to play in the future—discusses expected future HMO growth and important issues that will need to be considered as that growth occurs. The fifth section examines various methods of paying HMOs. The sixth section presents a summary of our analysis, while the final section sets forth recommendations regarding how to promote HMO growth without jeopardizing quality of care.

Table 7.1. **Profile of HMOs by Model Type, March 1988**

Model	Number	Percent	Change in Number, 1985–88 (%)	Enrollment		Change in Enrollment, 1985–88 (%)
				Number	Percent	
Staff	67	10	+22	3,737,617	12	+39
Group	68	10	+4	7,967,841	26	+23
Network	101	16	+17	6,138,536	20	+21
IPA	412	64	+128	13,171,431	43	+183
Total	648		+65	31,015,425		+64

Source: Interstudy 1988.
Note: Numbers do not include 543,690 HMO enrollees who have selected "open-ended" options.

Types of HMOs

The term "health maintenance organization" was coined in 1970 by Paul Elwood as part of a strategy to win Nixon administration support and congressional approval for prepaid health care as an alternative to the traditional FFS system (Strumpf 1981). The term was designed not only to improve the political viability of HMOs but also to emphasize the positive, prevention (health maintenance) focus of this alternative form of health care delivery (Decker 1981).

As they exist today, HMOs are organizations that assume contractual responsibility for providing a stated range of health care services to an enrolled population on a prepaid, capitation basis. Four different HMO models—staff, group, network, and independent practice associations (IPAs)—can be defined based on the way physician services are organized and the method by which physicians are paid. Staff, group, and network model HMOs are often collectively referred to as prepaid group practices (PGPs).

Staff model HMOs employ physicians on a full-time basis. While staff model HMOs, like all HMOs, are at risk financially for the services they provide, neither the physicians nor other personnel employed by the staff model HMO are at risk personally. As of March 1988, 10 percent of all U.S. HMO enrollees were enrolled in staff model HMOs (see tables 7.1 and 7.2). The Cigna HealthPlans of California, with 457,816 enrollees in March 1988, is the nation's largest staff model HMO (see table 7.3).

In group model arrangements, the HMO provides the facility, the nonphysician clinical staff, and administrative support and contracts with one large, multispecialty medical group practice for physician services. The HMO pays the physician group a fixed capitation fee for caring for

Table 7.2. HMO Enrollment and Number of Plans by Type of HMO, 1981–1987

HMO	1981	1983	1985	1987
	Enrollment			
Staff	1,137,332	2,145,072	2,685,875	3,707,553
Group	6,702,370	6,286,369	6,488,406	7,672,726
Network	844,795	2,170,579	5,073,011	5,865,832
IPA	1,581,675	1,888,760	4,646,315	12,039,909
Total	10,266,172	12,490,780	18,893,607	29,286,020
	Number of Plans			
Staff	44	59	55	69
Group	88	86	71	70
Network	21	36	86	100
IPA	90	99	181	411
Total	243	280	393	650

Sources: Interstudy 1985a, 1985b.

each HMO member each month. Physicians practicing in group model HMOs may enter into various profit-sharing arrangements that generally are not available to physicians in staff model systems (Rosenberg and Mackie 1981). Many of the larger group model HMOs own and operate their own hospitals. The Kaiser Foundation Health Plan in Northern California, with over 2.1 million enrollees in 1988, is the largest group model HMO. Nationwide, group model HMOs claimed 26 percent of total HMO enrollment in 1988 (Interstudy 1988).

Network model HMOs contract with more than one physician group. In contrast to group model HMOs, network model HMOs are supplied facilities and support personnel by the physician groups. Each physician group in the network receives a capitation payment for caring for enrollees who choose to receive care from that group. Most groups continue to see non-HMO patients in addition to HMO enrollees. The Health Net Plan of California, the largest network model HMO, served over 544,000 enrollees in March 1988 under a network arrangement. In 1988 there were 101 network HMOs with 6.1 million members, 20 percent of total HMO enrollees (Interstudy 1988).

The fourth type of HMO model is the individual practice association. In an IPA arrangement, the HMO utilizes a percentage of many practitioners' time to provide care to prepaid clients. In contrast to the network model, the IPA model HMO typically contracts with a large number of solo practitioners as well as single- or multispecialty group practices.

Table 7.3. The Ten Largest HMOs, March 1988

Name	Model	Profit Status[a]	March 1988 Enrollment
1. Kaiser Foundation Health Plan, Northern California	Group	NP	2,126,357
2. Kaiser Foundation Health Plan, Southern California	Group	NP	1,892,171
3. Health Insurance Plan of Greater New York	Group	NP	892,853
4. Health Net of California	Network	NP	544,861
5. HMO of Pennsylvania	IPA	P	502,800
6. Cigna Healthplans of California	Staff	P	457,816
7. Harvard Community Health Plan of Massachusetts	Network	NP	367,747
8. Maxicare of Southern California	IPA	P	363,491
9. Group Health Cooperative, Puget Sound, Washington	Staff	NP	339,075
10. Kaiser Foundation Health Plan of the Northwest, Oregon	Group	NP	342,622
Total			7,811,793
Total as percentage of total U.S. HMO enrollment			25%

Source: Interstudy 1988.
[a]NP = not-for-profit; P = for-profit.

Some HMOs contract with local physician associations, which then contract with individual physicians. The financial arrangements between the HMO and the physician contractors within an IPA model are complex and varied. Most IPA model HMOs reimburse their physicians based on agreed-upon fee schedules or payment limits drawn from a collective account (Friedland 1981).

Compared with PGPs, IPAs tend to have a greater number of participating physicians and a greater dispersion of delivery sites. These features provide IPA enrollees greater flexibility in choosing a physician. On the other hand, the existence of scattered private offices rather than a central facility limits opportunities for professional peer interaction in IPA model HMOs. Less physician loyalty to the HMO is likely, since IPA physicians can contract with several HMOs and HMO enrollees may constitute only a small percentage of any IPA physician's practice. There is thus uncertainty about whether IPAs can cut costs as effectively as other models of HMOs. Nonetheless, 64 percent of 648 HMO plans in

1988 were operating under an IPA model, and IPAs cared for 43 percent of total HMO enrollees. The HMO of Pennsylvania, the largest IPA, had an enrollment of over 502,000 in March 1988 (Interstudy 1988).

Since 1986 some HMOs, regardless of their model type, have offered their members an "open-ended" enrollment option in which enrollees are not required to use the HMO's participating providers and may enroll or disenroll at any time. Although enrollees are covered for services received outside of the HMO's provider network, benefits for services received outside of the HMO network are usually less comprehensive than the HMO benefits and often include deductibles, copayments, and/ or coinsurance. An HMO that provides an open-ended option thus offers increased flexibility to enrollees. As of March 1988, 47 HMOs operating in twenty-three states reported open-ended membership, with a total of 543,690 enrollees choosing this option (Interstudy 1988).

The Evolution of HMOs, 1970–1988

Federal Policies Encouraging HMO Growth

During the early 1970s, in an effort to slow the growth of health care expenditures, the federal government undertook measures to promote prepaid practice. The prepaid practice concept was incorporated into national legislation with the enactment of the Health Maintenance Organization Act of 1973 (PL 93–222). The key provisions of this legislation included establishment of a program of grants and loans to assist HMO development and requirements for federal qualification, including:

- requirements relating to the organizational structure of HMOs, including requirements for enrollee representation on an HMO's policymaking board, a program for resolution of enrollee grievances, and a quality assurance program;

- financial requirements to assure the fiscal solvency of HMOs;

- enrollment requirements, including requirements that no individual may be expelled from or refused enrollment in an HMO because of his health status and that the membership of an HMO be representative of the age, social, and income groups in the area it serves;

- requirements relating to the basic health services offered, including physician services, inpatient and outpatient hospital services and emergency services, short-term mental health services, referral services, diagnostic services, home health and preventive services, social services, and health education services;

- the pricing of HMO benefit packages using a community rating method;

- mandatory dual-choice option requirements for employers with twenty-five or more employees (employers with twenty-five or more employees were required to offer an HMO option to their employees if asked to by a federally qualified HMO in their geographic area) (L. D. Brown 1983; Mackie 1981; "Title XIII" 1982).

Through this legislation, and amendments to it in 1976 and 1978, which relaxed the requirements for federal qualification and increased the availability of federal funds, the federal government provided $145 million in grants and $219 million in loans between 1973 and 1983 for the development of 115 HMOs. The private sector invested an additional $253 million in HMOs between 1974 and 1980. Not all of the HMOs have been successful; failures have resulted in defaults on $42 million in federal loans (Iglehart 1984b).

The federal government stopped providing new grants to HMOs in 1981 (Iglehart 1984b). Since then, federal policy has focused on promotion of competition generally, incentives designed to increase private sector involvement in HMO development, and risk contracts to HMOs that agree to enroll Medicare beneficiaries. The federal government continues to designate HMOs that meet certain standards as federally qualified. In 1988 the 52 percent of HMOs that were federally qualified served approximately 80 percent of all HMO enrollees (Interstudy 1988).

Medicare and Medicaid Policies toward HMO Enrollment

Despite providing strong political and financial support for the growth of HMOs for the private sector, the federal government has moved comparatively slowly in formulating policies to encourage Medicare and Medicaid beneficiaries to enroll in prepaid health plans. This cautious approach has resulted in part from congressional concerns about the incentives of prepaid providers to underserve beneficiaries and the fact that inaccurate payment methods could allow HMOs to receive excessive profits. As a result, the federal government has exerted tighter control over reimbursement to, and the benefit packages and structural characteristics of, HMOs that enroll Medicare and Medicaid beneficiaries compared with those HMOs that do not.

Medicare

HMO involvement in serving Medicare beneficiaries was minimal prior to enactment of the 1972 amendments to the Social Security Act. Because of congressional reluctance to pay HMOs on the basis of prospectively determined capitation rates, even the 1972 amendments that authorized Medicare to reimburse HMOs on the basis of cost-based or risk contracts retained the essential features of cost reimbursement (Iglehart 1985b).

Cost-based contracts for Medicare enrollees in HMOs employed the usual Medicare cost principles for reimbursement. At the year's end, reasonable costs incurred by the HMO were reconciled with actual payments to it on behalf of Medicare enrollees. This year-end reconciliation ran counter to the fundamental principles upon which HMOs operated and undermined the cost-saving incentives of participating HMOs. Moreover, Medicare beneficiaries were not "locked in" to a single HMO for their care but could be reimbursed for services they received outside the HMO. HMOs thus lacked both the incentive and a mechanism for achieving control over Medicare beneficiaries' utilization.

Payments to HMOs under risk contracts were based on the adjusted average per capita cost (AAPCC). The AAPCC is an estimate of what the average cost of providing services to enrolled beneficiaries would be in the FFS sector. If the actual costs incurred by the HMO were lower than its AAPCC, it was allowed to share the savings equally with Medicare, up to a maximum HMO share of 10 percent of the AAPCC. If the HMO's costs were higher than the AAPCC, however, it had to absorb the entire loss. Risk-based contracts were only open to HMOs with at least two years' operating experience and a minimum enrollment of 25,000 (GAO 1986).

Few HMOs were willing to serve Medicare beneficiaries under these arrangements. As of July 1980 the Medicare program had signed thirty-eight cost contracts and one risk contract with HMOs covering approximately 61,500 Medicare enrollees (less than 1 percent of Medicare beneficiaries) (Trieger, Galblum, and Riley 1981). Recognizing the cost-saving potential of HMOs, the Carter administration worked aggressively to encourage the development of an HMO option for Medicare beneficiaries. Its legislative proposals were not enacted by Congress, however.

In an effort to develop reimbursement mechanisms more consistent with HMOs' usual method of operation, the Department of Health and Human Services initiated several HMO demonstration projects (Trieger, Galblum, and Riley 1981). Many of the restrictions on risk-based HMO contracts contained in Section 1876 were relaxed in the demonstration projects. Under the first part of the demonstration, contracts were awarded to six HMOs. HMOs were reimbursed at 95 percent of a prospectively adjusted AAPCC without retrospective adjustments. HMOs were required, however, to use any "profits" they realized to reduce cost sharing or to expand benefits for beneficiaries.

In 1982, under pressure to control federal health expenditures, Congress incorporated several provisions affecting HMOs into Section 114 of the Tax Equity and Fiscal Responsibility Act (Iglehart 1985b). The first provision expanded the definition of organizations eligible to contract with Medicare for care of Medicare beneficiaries to include Competitive

Medical Plans (CMPs). Unlike HMOs, CMPs are allowed to experience-rate their premiums based on enrollees' prior health care utilization and to impose deductibles (GAO 1986). The second TEFRA provision established risk-based contracts for HMOs without retroactive adjustments. In addition, TEFRA permitted Medicare to contract with HMOs whose enrollment was as low as 5,000 as long as no more than 50 percent of enrollees were eligible for Medicare or Medicaid.

Each risk-based HMO is required to calculate an adjusted community rate (ACR) prospectively. The ACR represents the premium an organization would charge its non-Medicare members for a benefit package of Medicare-covered services (including the organization's usual allowance for generating a surplus). The difference between the AAPCC paid by Medicare and the ACR is to be used to give Medicare beneficiaries additional benefits or decreased cost sharing (Iglehart 1985b).

TEFRA did not require that the HMO amendments become effective until the Department of Health and Human Services was reasonably certain that an appropriate payment methodology had been developed to assure actuarial equivalency between HMO and non-HMO members. Consequently, the final regulations were not issued until January 1985. In response to concerns about the quality of care that might be provided to Medicare beneficiaries by HMOs participating in risk contracts, Congress included a provision in the 1985 Consolidated Omnibus Reconciliation Act (COBRA) requiring PROs to scrutinize services furnished by HMOs and competitive medical plans under a Medicare risk-sharing contract as well as an HCFA review of all marketing materials (Ellwood 1986). By December 1986, 149 TEFRA risk contracts were in effect. These contracts covered four-fifths of the 3.5 percent of Medicare beneficiaries enrolled in HMOs as of December 1986 (McMillan, Lubitz, and Russell 1987). By January 1988, 981,145 Medicare beneficiaries (an increase from 2.8 percent of the total to 3 percent) were enrolled in TEFRA risk-contracting programs (Rossiter and Langwell 1988). The highest concentrations of enrolled beneficiaries are in Florida, Minnesota, and California (see table 7.4).

Medicaid

As enacted in 1965, Title XIX did not provide for enrollment of Medicaid beneficiaries in HMOs. Section 1902 of the 1967 amendments to the Social Security Act gave states legislative authority to contract with HMOs but assured Medicaid beneficiaries freedom to obtain medical care from any qualified provider willing to serve them (Trieger, Galblum, and Riley 1981). The amendments specified the following guidelines:

- States must specify the amount of the premium, the services covered, and the term of the contract.

Table 7.4. **TEFRA Risk Contracts and Enrollees, December 1986**

State	Number of Contracts	Number of Enrollees	TEFRA Risk Enrollees as Percentage of Total Medicare Beneficiaries in State
Florida	11	175,192	9.0
California	14	164,296	5.9
Minnesota	11	137,390	25.6
Illinois	7	53,525	3.8
Massachusetts	15	51,509	6.5
Michigan	12	38,550	3.5
Pennsylvania	4	21,296	1.2
Oregon	2	21,221	5.8
Hawaii	3	17,653	18.2
New York	7	16,681	0.7
Nevada	3	14,970	15.3
New Jersey	5	14,246	1.4
Kansas	12	13,371	4.0
New Mexico	4	12,605	8.8
Arizona	1	11,420	2.9
Colorado	5	11,396	3.9
Indiana	2	9,906	1.5
Oklahoma	3	4,285	1.1
Ohio	5	3,312	0.2
Nebraska	1	3,244	1.5
Maryland	3	2,681	0.6
Iowa	1	2,600	0.6
Rhode Island	1	2,506	1.7
Connecticut	1	2,422	0.6
Tennessee	1	2,361	0.4
Texas	6	1,900	0.1
Wisconsin	3	1,759	0.3
South Carolina	1	938	0.3
North Carolina	1	377	Less than 0.1
Missouri	1	139	Less than 0.1
Utah	2	1	Less than 0.1
Georgia	1	0	0
Total	149	813,712	

Total Number of Medicare Enrollees in the U.S.   29,421,000
TEFRA Enrollees as Percentage of Medicare Population   2.8%

Source: McMillan, Lubitz, and Russell 1987.

- Payment of the premium fully discharges the state from responsibility for the cost of covered benefits.
- The premium amount and the covered benefits should be renegotiated periodically.
- The HMO must provide the state with data to comply with federal reporting requirements.

Within these general guidelines, states had a great deal of flexibility in signing and monitoring HMO contracts. Between 1971 and 1973 twelve states signed sixty-six contracts with HMOs to serve 371,000 Medicaid beneficiaries. Fifty of these were implemented in California, where a massive enrollment of beneficiaries into prepaid health plans (PHPs) was undertaken. Unfortunately, this rapid growth was not adequately monitored. Serious complaints about cost, quality, enrollment practices, and corporate accountability were raised within a year as plans in California exploited the Medicaid population. The resulting scandal led to congressional hearings in 1975, with the outcome that regulations governing enrollment of Medicaid beneficiaries in PHPs were tightened. Some of the key regulations deriving from the 1975 hearings include the following: states were given control over enrollment and disenrollment procedures; HMOs were required to make services available twenty-four hours per day, seven days a week; and HMOs were required to establish an internal grievance procedure and an adequate medical record-keeping system (Trieger, Galblum, and Riley 1981).

Further restrictions were incorporated in the HMO amendments of 1976 to prevent the scandals in California from recurring. Federal matching funds were limited to federally qualified HMOs (none of the PHPs in California had been federally qualified), with few exceptions, and enrollment of Medicaid and Medicare beneficiaries was limited to 50 percent of membership. The effect of this increased regulation was to lower the percentage of Medicaid beneficiaries enrolled in HMOs. By 1980 only 270,000 Medicaid beneficiaries, representing 2 percent of eligibles, were enrolled in fifty-three HMOs in seventeen states (Trieger, Galblum, and Riley 1981).

By 1981 attitudes had changed appreciably. The HMO concept was much more established. States were facing increasing pressure to lower costs, and the legislative trend was toward decreased federal monitoring. The 1981 OBRA amendments, therefore, moved away from the above restrictions and allowed states increased flexibility in financing and delivering health services in their Medicaid programs. States were permitted to establish their own quality standards for HMOs. HMOs contracting with Medicaid were permitted to have a Medicare and Medicaid enrollment of up to 75 percent. Waivers of federal Medicaid regulations were authorized to permit states to establish primary care case management systems for their Medicaid programs and to select providers based on their cost-effectiveness (Neuschler 1985a).

As of August 1984 twenty-five states had applied for waivers to restrict the freedom of choice of Medicaid beneficiaries to a defined set of providers. Most states sought to implement these waivers under a primary care case management system. HMOs may participate under the waivers as primary care case managers. A number of states, including New Jersey, Delaware, and Iowa, are aggressively pursuing enrollment of Medicaid beneficiaries in HMOs. Wisconsin has gone even further, requiring the AFDC population in Dane and Milwaukee counties to choose among state-approved HMOs (Rowland and Lyons 1987). Except under special circumstances, beneficiaries may not receive care on a fee-for-service basis; a beneficiary may, however, change HMOs.

By December 1986, 802,750 Medicaid recipients were enrolled in 125 HMOs in twenty-five states and the District of Columbia. Medicaid enrollment in HMOs is concentrated in older and larger plans, with over 67 percent of enrollees in HMOs that are at least ten years old and over 50 percent in plans with over 50,000 members (Gruber, Shadle, and Polich 1988).

Growth of HMOs

In 1971, prior to the national HMO legislation, there were thirty HMOs in the United States which together enrolled three million members (OHMO 1983). As of March 1988 the number of HMOs had grown to 648, with an enrollment of over 31 million (Interstudy 1988). Between 1981 and 1987 the average annual rate of increase in HMO enrollment was 18.5 percent (Gruber, Shadle, and Polich 1988). Total HMO enrollment increased by 36 percent in 1986 and by 14 percent in 1987. The number of HMO plans increased by 16.9 percent per year for the years 1981–87 (Interstudy 1988). By the end of March 1988 an estimated 12.8 percent of the U.S. population was enrolled in HMOs (see fig. 7.1). Since 1980, enrollment growth rates have been highest for HMOs that have been in existence for fewer than five years, for IPA model HMOs, and for HMOs with 50,000–100,000 members (Interstudy 1985a, 1988). In March 1988 the ten largest HMOs claimed 25 percent of the total HMO enrollment (see table 7.3).

Recent Trends in the HMO Market

Affiliations among HMOs have been increasing in recent years. The number of HMOs operated under common ownership or common management or through a common marketing or membership office grew from 99 in 1981 to 156 in 1984. During this period enrollment in affiliated HMOs

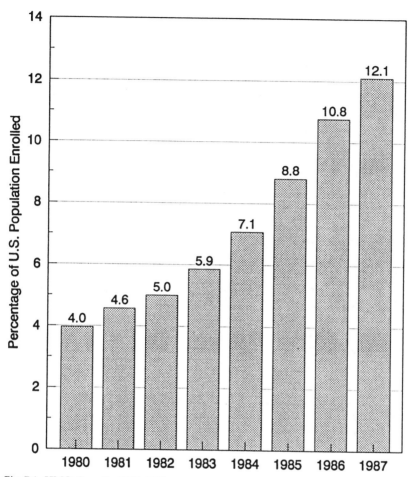

Fig. 7.1. **HMO Growth, 1980–1987**
(*Source:* Interstudy 1988; DHHS 1988.)

increased by 75 percent to 10.9 million (McNamara-Bennett 1985; OHMO 1983; Whitney 1985). In 1983 the 127 HMOs in affiliations were owned and operated by thirteen national firms and accounted for 46 percent of all HMOs. By December 1986 there were 310 affiliated plans owned and operated by forty-two national firms and claiming 60 percent of all HMO enrollees (Gruber, Shadle, and Polich 1988; OHMO 1985a; Whitney 1985). In 1988 Kaiser Foundation Health Plans, with twelve HMO affiliates and over 5 million enrollees, had the largest enrollment of all HMO chains (see table 7.5) (Gruber, Shadle, and Polich 1988).

Table 7.5. **The Five Largest Multistate HMO Chains, January 1988**

Name	Number of Plans	Enrollment, January 1988
1. Kaiser Foundation Health Plans	12	5,233,370
2. Maxicare Health Plans	33	2,216,155
3. CIGNA Healthplan	27	1,236,667
4. United Healthcare	27	1,017,116
5. Health Insurance Plan of Greater New York	3	969,757

Source: Interstudy 1988.

The number of for-profit HMOs also has been increasing. Until recently the HMO industry was predominantly not-for-profit. In December 1982, 49 (18 percent) of 269 HMOs were for-profit entities (Whitney 1985); by March 1988, 433 (67 percent) of 648 HMOs were for-profit (Interstudy 1988). Interstudy projects that if present growth trends continue, over 50 percent of HMO members will be enrolled in for-profit plans by December 1988 (Interstudy 1988).

Among for-profit HMOs there has been an increase over the past few years in the number of publicly owned HMOs. Prior to 1983 no HMO firms were publicly owned (Iglehart 1984b). In February 1983 U.S. Health Care Systems became the first HMO firm to offer publicly traded stock. By May 1984 there were seven publicly owned HMO companies (Alex Brown & Sons 1984; Traska 1985b). In 1985 six additional HMO companies offered publicly traded stocks, bringing the total number of publicly owned HMO companies to thirteen (Sherlock 1986; Whitney 1985). By the end of 1986 the total number of publicly owned HMOs had increased to fifteen (Alex Brown & Sons, 1986).

Characteristics of HMO Enrollees

Although HMOs had enrolled about 13 percent of the U.S. population by the end of 1987 (see fig. 7.1), enrollees were not demographically representative of the population as a whole. According to Berki and Ashcraft's (1980) review of the literature, HMO enrollees are more likely to be married than single. A 1984 Louis Harris and Associates survey conducted for the Henry J. Kaiser Family Foundation reported that 66 percent of HMO enrollees were less than forty years of age. The Harris survey also revealed that middle-income ($15,001–25,000) and white-collar households, as well as households insured through a family member employed in a large company, were more likely to report an HMO membership in 1984 than in 1980. In 1984, 9 percent of privately insured households nationwide reported at least one family member who be-

Table 7.6. The Top Ten States Ranked by Percentage of Population Enrolled in HMOs, March 1988

State	Estimated Percentage of Population Enrolled in HMOs*	Number of HMO Enrollees (millions)	Percentage Change in Enrollment, June 1986–March 1988
California	28.5	7.68	+19
Wisconsin	22.3	1.07	+15
Massachusetts	21.9	1.28	+32
Hawaii	20.8	.22	+13
Minnesota	20.7	.87	−17
Oregon	20.0	.54	+26
Rhode Island	19.4	.19	+23
Colorado	18.9	.62	+50
Connecticut	17.6	.56	+78
Arizona	17.2	.57	+28

Sources: The estimated percentages of the population enrolled in HMOs were calculated from Census 1986; the number of HMO enrollees is taken from Interstudy 1988.

longed to an HMO, compared with 6 percent in 1980 (Louis Harris and Associates 1984).

As of March 1988 California had more HMO enrollees than any other state (see table 7.6) (Interstudy 1988). By 1988 HMOs claimed 20 percent or more of the population in six states (Interstudy 1988). HMO penetration varied across metropolitan areas, however: 36 percent in San Francisco, 32 percent in Minneapolis, 27 percent in Los Angeles, and 24 percent in Portland, for example (National Industrial Council for HMO Development 1984).

In January 1988 there were approximately 981,000 Medicare beneficiaries enrolled in HMOs, representing 3 percent of all Medicare beneficiaries (Rossiter and Langwell 1988; Wood 1988). Overall, Medicare beneficiaries constitute 3.2 percent of all HMO enrollees. In December 1986 some 3.6 percent of Medicaid beneficiaries were enrolled in HMOs (Gruber, Shadle, and Polich 1988; Parker 1988). Medicaid beneficiaries constitute 3 percent of all HMO enrollees (Gruber, Shadle, and Polich 1988; Interstudy 1988).

No consistent or definitive evidence has been reported that proves that individuals who join HMOs are healthier than those who remain in FFS sector. Several investigators have compared the utilization of HMO enrollees and nonenrollees, however. For example, HMO enrollees have been reported to have lower preenrollment rates of utilization than their FFS counterparts (Berki and Ashcraft 1980; Blumberg 1980; Gaus, Cooper, and Hirschman 1981; Hellinger 1987; Luft 1981). In addition, prior to enrolling in an HMO, HMO enrollees averaged 53 percent fewer inpatient days than those retaining FFS coverage (470 days per 1,000 versus 994 days per 1,000). Whether this lower rate of utilization was a reflection of better health or unmet need was unclear (Jackson-Beeck and Kleinman, 1983). Luft reported that individuals who chose to enroll in HMOs were less likely to have a strong tie to a physician than non-HMO enrollees (Luft 1981). A strong tie to a physician may be a marker for a sicker individual. The 1984 Louis Harris survey reported that HMO members and nonmembers were comparable in terms of a number of measures of health status: incidence of chronic illness in the family (12 percent of HMO members reported that at least one family member had a chronic illness, compared with 9 percent of nonmembers); days spent in bed due to illness in the previous twelve months (49 percent of HMO members reported none, compared with 50 percent of nonmembers); and self-reported health status (53 percent of HMO members reported excellent health, compared with 57 percent of nonmembers) (Louis Harris and Associates 1984). A recent review of the literature by Hellinger suggests that the health status of HMO enrollees is approximately the same as that of enrollees in traditional health plans (Hellinger 1987).

Rates of Disenrollment from HMOs

The Office of Health Maintenance Organizations, or OHMO (now called the Office of Prepaid Health Care) reported that in 1985, 5 percent of those enrolled in federally qualified HMOs terminated their membership in the HMO in which they were enrolled (OHMO 1985a). Recently reported rates of disenrollment from a few HMOs have ranged from 6 percent to 20 percent (DesHarnais 1985; Lewis 1984; Mechanic, Weiss, and Cleary 1983; Sorenson and Wersinger 1981). Recently reported disenrollment rates may be quite misleading, however. HMOs, for example, typically record as terminations not only voluntary terminations (members who choose to disenroll from the HMO to enroll in another form of health coverage) but also involuntary terminations (members who disenroll because of job loss or relocation) and changes in coverage within the same HMO (Mechanic, Weiss, and Cleary 1983). Mechanic has found that the disparity between the reported disenrollment rate and the number of real terminations (voluntary and involuntary) in one large staff model HMO was about 7 percent. Mechanic also found that in addition to tending to be dissatisfied with their access to care in the HMO, disenrollees had fewer health problems and were less likely to have established a stable relationship with an HMO physician who was available when needed than was the case for continuing HMO members. Use of a non-HMO physician in the preceding year was the strongest identified predictor of disenrollment (Mechanic, Weiss, and Cleary 1983). In general, studies have shown that utilization of services was lower for HMO dis-enrollees than for HMO enrollees who chose to remain in the HMO. However, in comparison to FFS patients, HMO disenrollees had either higher health care use or higher health care costs after leaving the HMO (Luft and Miller 1988).

Do HMOs Save Money?

One of the most important issues in assessing the value and future impact of HMOs is whether they save money. In contrast to the situation for FFS providers, the revenue going to HMOs does not increase as more services are provided to patients. The presumption therefore exists that HMOs will provide care at less cost than FFS providers will. The collection of data to substantiate this presumption, however, has been complicated by difficulties in ensuring the comparability of patient characteristics and quality of care in HMOs versus the FSS system. Nonetheless, substantial data do exist that suggest that HMOs in the past have provided health care at a lower total cost than did FFS providers.

Total Costs

Luft, in his extensive review of the literature, examined six studies per-formed between 1962 and 1976 that compared total annual health costs for people enrolled in HMO and non-HMO plans (Luft 1981). Each of the studies found that total annual costs per person (i.e., premium plus additional out-of-pocket expenses) were 10–40 percent lower for members of prepaid group practice HMOs than for non-HMO enrollees (Luft 1978, 1981). Luft cautioned that because of differences in the populations stud-ied, observed differences in the cost of care might not reflect lower cost-patterns of practice.

More recently, the Rand Corporation reported that HMO enrollees generated 25 percent lower annual expenditures per person than did individuals in the FFS sector (Manning et al. 1984). The Rand study compared cost and usage among people randomly assigned to one of three payment plans: free FFS; FFS with patient cost sharing; or a prepaid group practice (the Group Health Cooperative of Puget Sound). The study also compared a sample of self-selected prepaid group practice members with the other three groups. The study demonstrated that the average annual cost of providing medical services in the HMO was $439 per person, compared with $609 per person in the free FFS setting. Within the free FFS group, 85 percent of enrollees used some medical services over the course of the year, and 11 percent had one or more hospital-izations. In the HMO group 87 percent used at least some medical service, but only 7 percent were hospitalized. The total number of hospital days was greater for FFS members: 83 days per 100 persons, compared with 49 days per 100 persons for HMO members. These lower hospital utilization rates accounted for the 25 percent lower costs for HMO enrollees compared with FFS enrollees (Manning et al. 1984). A more recent survey performed by the Group Health Association of America (GHAA), a trade association of HMOs, found that the total number of hospital days for FFS members continues to be higher than that for HMO members: 96 days per 100 persons, compared with 46 days for HMO members (GHAA 1988c).

The Rate of Increase in Premiums

Luft has reported that among federal government employees between 1961 and 1974 premiums grew at an annual rate of 9.5 percent for those enrolled in prepaid group practices, compared with 10.4 percent for FFS enrollees (Luft 1980, 1981). Factors accounting for changes in the premiums over time were not clear. OHMO also has reported that between 1980 and 1982 the rate of growth in HMO premiums was lower than the rate of growth in traditional insurance premiums (OHMO 1983). Newhouse, in contrast, reported that between 1976 and 1981 premiums of HMO enrollees for a two-adult, two-child family increased by 74 percent, compared with a 75 percent increase in per capita health care costs nationally for individuals under sixty-five years of age (Newhouse et al. 1985).

According to a recent marketing research report, the average premiums charged by HMOs increased 15–17 percent per year between 1982 and 1983, compared with an average increase in premiums for traditional health insurance during the same period of 21–23 percent per year. The report also stated that many HMOs now offer premiums at prices comparable to or lower than those charged by indemnity plans (Alex Brown & Sons 1984). Interstudy reported that in 1984 HMO premiums had increased by 10 percent from the previous year to an average family premium of $189 per month (Interstudy 1985a). From 1985 to 1986, average HMO premium increases were under 3 percent (GHAA 1988a). Between 1986 and 1987 both HMO and traditional health insurance premiums increased at a modest rate, 3–4 percent (Gabel et al. 1988).

The Rate of Increase in Costs

Despite the lower rate of increase in premiums charged by HMOs, the rate of growth in costs per HMO enrollee is only slightly lower than the rate of growth in costs per FFS enrollee. Luft examined changes in cost for HMO enrollees from several sources (the Federal Employees Health Benefits Program, the California state employees, and Kaiser-Oregon members) between 1960 and 1974 and found that the rate of growth in total costs was only slightly lower for HMO enrollees than for FFS enrollees. Luft did find, however, that although HMO and FFS enrollees had similar rates of increase in health care costs, HMO enrollees' total costs were lower than those of FFS enrollees at any point in time (Luft 1980, 1981). More recently, Newhouse analyzed data from 1976–81 and found that the rates of increase in costs in HMOs were comparable to the rates of increase in personal medical expenditures in the nation as a whole (Newhouse et al. 1985). Personal medical expenditures are dominated by figures for the FFS system.

How Have HMOs Lowered Costs?

The 1984 Rand study reported 40 percent fewer admissions and 40 percent fewer hospital days for HMO enrollees than for those in the free FFS plan. HMO enrollees were also 5–20 percent less likely to be admitted than were those in the cost-sharing FFS group (Manning et al. 1984). The Rand study reported 8.4 admissions and 49 hospital days per 100 persons per year for HMO enrollees, compared with 13.8 annual admissions and 83 hospital days per 100 persons per year among FFS enrollees (Gaus, Cooper, and Hirschman 1981). The Rand findings are thus consistent with Luft's earlier report, based on a review of the literature, which found that hospital admission rates for HMO enrollees were as much as 40 percent lower per year than those for enrollees in FFS plans (Luft 1981). More recently, the GHAA has reported that inpatient utilization rates for HMO enrollees are substantially below national averages. For patients under age sixty-five, HMO members had an annual average of 35 hospital days per 100 persons in 1986, whereas the national average was 61 hospital days per 100 persons. For patients sixty-five or older, HMO enrollees had an annual average of 184 hospital days per 100 persons in 1986, while the national average was 312 hospital days per 100 persons (GHAA 1988c).

In comparing hospital admission rates for HMO and FFS patients, Siu et al. (1988) found that the rate of discretionary surgery was lower in the HMO setting, whereas the rate of nondiscretionary surgery was the same in the HMO and FFS sectors. The authors concluded that the reduced rates of hospitalization seen in the HMO setting did not occur across the board; rather, discretionary surgery was selectively avoided in the HMO setting.

In a much smaller-scale study of a limited patient population, Yelin found no significant differences in hospital utilization rates between rheumatoid arthritis (RA) patients cared for by rheumatologists in HMOs and patients cared for by rheumatologists in fee-for-service practices. No significant differences were observed in the per capita number of hospital admissions for RA, the length of stay of admissions for RA, or the number of per capita hospital days for treatment of RA (Yelin et al. 1985).

Arnould examined differences in resource use in patients undergoing four types of surgery in HMOs and in FFS practices and found that the full cost of hospital stays was significantly lower for HMO patients only in the case of appendectomies. Total costs for appendectomies were $891 (35 percent) lower per case in HMOs than in FFS patients. No differences in total hospital cost were found between HMO and FFS patients admitted for cholecystectomy, hernia repair, or hysterectomy (Arnould, Debrock, and Pollard 1984).

The differences in costs for HMO and FFS enrollees have not been related to consistent differences in outpatient service utilization. The Rand study found no difference between HMO and FFS enrollees in number of ambulatory care visits (Manning et al. 1984). In contrast, Yelin reported that HMO rheumatologists saw their patients less frequently than did FFS rheumatologists (3.47 fewer office visits per HMO patient over a one-year period) (Yelin et al. 1985). Although not addressed by Yelin, this difference may have been related to differences in referral and follow-up patterns between HMO and FFS generalists and specialists (Myerowitz 1985). No studies of rates of referrals to specialists in HMOs versus FFS practices have been reported. No evidence has emerged to demonstrate that differences in HMO and FFS costs are attributable to differences in the quality of care provided (see chapter 10).

The Future of HMOs

Enrollment

Several projections suggest that there will be continued growth in HMO enrollment in the future. A national study of forty HMOs conducted by Arthur D. Little, Inc. (1985), for example, predicted that HMOs would enroll 25–30 percent of the U.S. population by 1995, compared with 6 percent in 1984. More conservative observers predict a limit to potential enrollment of 60–70 million, or 20–25 percent of the population (Alex Brown & Sons 1986). The basis for these predictions is not clear. Our own case study of HMO development in Baltimore identified a widespread belief among informed observers that HMOs would capture no more than 30 percent of the Baltimore population by 1990 (Steinberg and Hynes 1986). Nonurban areas are unlikely to have substantial HMO enrollment. A total nationwide enrollment of 15–25 percent of the population by 1995 seems reasonable.

Several factors will influence the penetration of HMOs into the health care market. One of the most important factors will be the future strength of society's concerns about health care costs and its perceptions about the ability of HMOs compared with FFS providers to control them. If in response to the cost-conscious style of practice prevalent in HMOs, for example, FFS providers themselves become more cost-conscious, employers' and others' current attraction to HMOs may decrease.

Second, as our case study of HMO development in Baltimore demonstrated, local as well as national consumer attitudes will have a critical impact on the ultimate market share of HMOs. The HMO managers and other informed observers whom we interviewed, for example, believed that the conservative attitudes of the Baltimore population, the strength of the Baltimore population's loyalty to its neighborhood doctors, and a reluctance of individuals to forgo the freedom of choosing their own physician would limit Baltimore's ultimate interest in HMOs (Steinberg and Hynes 1986). Consistent with this view is the finding that nationwide the unwillingness of individuals not enrolled in HMOs to break existing ties with their physicians is one of the most significant obstacles to continued growth in HMO enrollment (Luft 1981). Nonetheless, a 1984 Louis Harris survey identified increased interest in HMO membership among eligible nonmembers (50 percent expressed interest in HMO membership in 1984, compared with 39 percent in 1980) and continued satisfaction on the part of HMO members with the services they receive (85 percent were satisfied with the services they had received in 1984, compared with 89 percent in 1980) (Louis Harris and Associates 1984).

Physician attitudes are a third major factor that will influence the future rate of growth of HMOs. Although the 1984 Louis Harris survey found increased participation in and acceptance of HMOs by physicians in 1984 compared with 1980, it also demonstrated a continued belief among physicians that the care offered by HMOs is inferior to that offered by FFS plans. The concerns of physicians were based on beliefs that HMOs perform fewer lab and diagnostic tests and employ less qualified physicians and that many HMOs do not allow for an adequate doctor-patient relationship. The same Harris survey found no evidence that HMO physicians were less skilled, as measured by board certification and length of time in practice, than the physician community as a whole, however. The survey also found that physicians in HMOs were less satisfied with their income than were FFS doctors but that they were more satisfied than FFS doctors with their professional peer support and the time available to them for nonprofessional interests (Louis Harris and Associates 1984).

These findings and sentiments have also emerged from two recent studies comparing physicians in HMOs with physicians in the FFS sector. One of these studies, conducted by Blue Cross/Blue Shield in North Carolina, analyzed why physicians in FFS practice choose to join a prepaid group practice. The investigators found that joiners believed they would control costs while maintaining quality, whereas nonjoiners saw the cost-controlling incentives of the plan as having a negative effect on the quality of care. Physicians who did not join prepaid plans had more established practices and a greater number of patients and had lived in the area for a longer time than those physicians who joined HMOs. Those physicians who joined the HMO reported smaller incomes than those who did not join (Dolan 1985).

In another survey of 154 physicians who had worked in eight New England HMOs, a comparison of physicians who stayed with the HMOs (stayers) with those who left (leavers) revealed that leavers had a significantly higher income in their new practice than stayers did in their HMO. Leavers reported working longer hours in their new practice than stayers reported working and cited the potential for greater autonomy as the most important factor in their decision to leave (Mick et al. 1983).

Fourth, the strength of future government support of HMO activities will influence the market share of HMOs in coming years. Regulations such as mandatory dual-choice requirements, which require employers with twenty-five or more employees to offer an HMO health insurance option if asked to, help HMOs gain inroads into the large-employee market. Increased efforts by state governments to enroll Medicaid beneficiaries in HMOs would also affect the magnitude of future HMO enrollment. If, for example, state governments were to mandate HMO enrollment for their Medicaid populations in an effort to gain control over their health care expenditures, the number and character of HMOs might change substantially. Our case study in Baltimore suggested that at least at this time, mandatory enrollment of Maryland's Medicaid beneficiaries in HMOs is unlikely (Steinberg and Hynes 1986). The primary reasons for this were concerns among legislators about the abridgment of the freedom of choice of Medicaid beneficiaries and the appearance of promotion of a two-tier medical care system. Wisconsin, however, has enrolled its entire AFDC-Medicaid population in HMOs (see chapter 6; and Rowland and Lyons 1987).

Finally, the future market share achieved by HMOs will be influenced by the competition HMOs experience from newer types of provider arrangements, such as PPOs. In contrast to HMOs, PPOs offer the prospect of cost control with few restrictions on enrollees' choice of physicians. PPOs also tend to be subject to less state regulation than HMOs. Informed observers interviewed in our case study of HMO development in Baltimore suggested that PPOs would likely enroll 15 percent or more of the Baltimore population by 1990 (Steinberg and Hynes 1986). Such strong competition from other forms of prepaid health care undoubtedly will limit the ultimate market share achieved by HMOs.

Other Issues

Our review of HMO growth over the past decade and our analysis of HMO development in Baltimore suggest several other issues pertinent to the future of HMOs that are worthy of consideration. The first is that whatever HMO enrollment is likely to be over the next several years, it is unlikely to be evenly distributed geographically. The attitudes and lifestyles of those living in certain parts of the country will limit the extent to which HMOs are able to establish themselves there. Conversely, certain demographic conditions will attract HMOs to an area. These include a population base of close to or more than 1 million, a high percentage of young working individuals, especially ones who are new arrivals to the area, and a concentration of employees in a few large firms at which marketing efforts can be directed at relatively low cost (Steinberg and Hynes 1986).

Second, the structure of the HMO industry has been changing in recent years. An increasing number of HMOs are becoming affiliated with chains or are merging, and an increasing proportion of HMOs are becoming for-profit enterprises. Two of the nation's five largest HMO chains (Maxicare Health Plans, Inc., and the United Healthcare Corporation), however, reported losses for fiscal year 1987 ($256 million and $16 million, respectively) (Gruber, Shadle, and Polich 1988). These trends bear watching, since they may significantly influence the conduct and performance of the HMO industry in the future.

Third, our case study of HMO development called attention to the fact that certain types of regulation of HMOs may be beneficial, while others, although well-intentioned, may create more problems than they solve. Since implementation of a capital reserve requirement for HMOs in Maryland, for example, there have been no HMO financial failures. In the late 1970s, prior to implementation of this regulation, in contrast, financial failures among HMOs were common in Baltimore. The requirement that at least 25–50 percent of the enrollees in an HMO that contracts with a state Medicaid agency must be neither Medicaid nor Medicare beneficiaries helps to assure that HMOs do not become Medicaid mills, but it may limit the ability of HMOs to undertake Medicaid contracts (Steinberg and Hynes, 1986). Such a requirement, which may be essential to assuring high-quality care in HMOs caring for Medicaid beneficiaries, may be difficult to fulfill in some circumstances given the locational requirements and marketing practices necessary to attract both Medicaid and non-Medicaid beneficiaries.

Fourth, given the financial incentives implicit in HMOs, there is a need to ensure that the quality of care received by all HMO enrollees is not eroded. Whether quality of care is best addressed through regulation, the competitive marketplace, or other means is as yet unclear.

A final important issue relates to the role HMOs are likely to play in caring for Medicaid and Medicare beneficiaries in the future. As budgetary pressures on state and federal governments increase, the desire of government officials to gain control over rising health care costs intensifies. Increased enrollment of Medicaid and Medicare beneficiaries in HMOs is seen as one potential vehicle for achieving such cost savings. At present only 3 percent of such beneficiaries are enrolled in HMOs. Some observers have questioned whether HMOs can be successful in controlling the costs of Medicaid beneficiaries. Medicaid beneficiaries, they argue, are sicker and have more pressing social problems than non-Medicaid beneficiaries and, given their lower level of education, will be harder to train in the cost-cutting utilization procedures practiced in HMOs. The general consensus among those whom we interviewed in Baltimore was that HMOs could achieve major cost savings in the care of Medicaid beneficiaries. We believe that states will increasingly adopt strategies to enroll Medicaid beneficiaries in prepaid forms of care such as HMOs. One strategy for doing so that is less stringent than mandatory enrollment requirements would be a financial incentive for Medicaid beneficiaries to enroll in HMOs (Steinberg and Hynes 1986). The future of Medicare beneficiary enrollment in HMOs is less clear and depends in large part, we believe, on development of an equitable methodology for determination of capitation premiums paid to HMOs for care of Medicare beneficiaries (Anderson et al. 1986b).

How Should HMOs Be Paid?

One major issue that will shape the future of HMOs is the development of payment rates that compensate HMOs fairly for the cost of caring for a defined patient population, that is, that do not lead to excess profits or create incentives to avoid patients who are poor health risks. Despite the importance of the capitation payment rate, however, relatively little attention has been given as yet by public payers, employers, or health services researchers to methods for establishing appropriate capitation payment rates (Anderson et al. 1986b).

Public payers such as Medicare and Medicaid, as well as private payers such as corporations, have two basic approaches available to them for establishing the rates they pay for their beneficiaries or employees who choose to enroll in HMOs: one approach is to act as a price giver, essentially setting the price they are willing to pay an HMO; the other is to act as a price taker, essentially relying on the HMO and the competitive marketplace to establish a fair payment rate. Several issues and concerns related to these alternative approaches are worthy of consideration.

Setting Payment Rates

The first issue is that all currently available methods for establishing capitation payment rates have major limitations. Currently, the HCFA pays HMOs that enroll Medicare beneficiaries 95 percent of the AAPCC of Medicare beneficiaries, an estimate of what the cost of treating Medicare beneficiaries is expected to be in the FFS sector. The AAPCC is derived by adjusting average national per capita Medicare costs for historical differences between national per capita costs and those in the county in which the HMO is located, as well as for the age, sex, welfare status, and institutional status of those Medicare beneficiaries who actually enroll in the HMO.

Several investigators have demonstrated that the AAPCC is a poor predictor of Medicare beneficiaries' subsequent utilization and expenditures (Beebe, Lubitz, and Eggers 1985; Hornbrook 1984). The current AAPCC probably explains no more than 1 percent of the variance in Medicare beneficiaries' annual expenditures. In addition, certain factors used in the creation of the AAPCC are not significant predictors of the variation in per capita expenditures among Medicare beneficiaries (Anderson et al. 1986a). Gender, for example, is not a significant predictor of per capita expenditures once other factors are taken into consideration. Other AAPCC factors have only a small explanatory power. Among the AAPCC variables, per capita expenditures in the county where the beneficiary lives represent the most statistically significant predictor of Medicare expenditures.

In addition to its limited predictive accuracy, the AAPCC has been criticized because (1) the institutional status variable used in its calculation is difficult to collect; (2) the geographic adjustment may perpetuate regional differences in health care costs that are based upon inefficient medical practices; (3) when there are a small number of Medicare beneficiaries living in a county, the AAPCC can lead to considerable variation in payment rates across county lines; and (4) the formula rewards certain behavior, such as institutionalization, without regard to the need for those practices (Anderson et al. 1986b).

In view of these limitations, several alternatives to the AAPCC methodology have been proposed. One of the most promising approaches is to incorporate an adjustment for individuals' prior utilization of health care resources into the AAPCC (Anderson and Knickman 1984; Beebe, Lubitz, and Eggers 1985). This is the only modification to the AAPCC that actually has been used to pay HMOs in a demonstration project.

Although this approach has the advantage of improving the predictive accuracy of the AAPCC, it has the disadvantage of basing future payment on past utilization rates without regard for the need or medical appropriateness of that past utilization. As a result, this method has been criticized for not providing appropriate incentives to providers (McClure 1984).

In response to this criticism, one possibility is to modify the payment methodology so that prior utilization information is incorporated into the AAPCC, but in such a way the degree of physician discretion involved in hospitalization decisions is taken into account. This can be done in a way that provides significantly better predictive accuracy than is available from the current AAPCC, and with little sacrifice in predictive accuracy compared with the use of the AAPCC adjusted for all types of prior utilization (Anderson et al. 1986a). This methodology is premised on the notion that hospitalization decisions involving little or only moderate physician discretion are more likely to be medically necessary than are those involving a high degree of physician discretion. Although this premise may be true, thus providing the virtue of not rewarding medical practices that are most likely to be unnecessary, the proposed adjustment for physician discretion has the disadvantage of underpaying providers in cases in which hospitalizations classified as highly discretionary are nevertheless medically appropriate.

An alternative to these types of prior-utilization adjustments is one in which the AAPCC is adjusted for self-reported or objectively determined health status. Thomas et al. (1984), for example, have shown that either subjective or objective adjustments for health status improve the predictive accuracy of the AAPCC. The data required to make these types of adjustments would be considerable, however; and they would potentially be subject to biased reporting as well as difficulties in preserving the confidentiality of individuals' medical histories.

The alternative to rate-setting approaches is to rely on competition within the marketplace to establish capitation payment rates that are actuarially fair and provide physicians with strong incentives to practice cost-effective medicine. It is this competitive approach that the private sector has relied upon to establish payment rates for HMO enrollees. From the perspective of a payer with considerable monopsony power, such as Medicare, the major disadvantage of a market-determined payment rate is that it will be costlier than one that it establishes and offers to HMOs in a "take it or leave it" fashion.

Problems When Rates Are Not Set Appropriately

Having described the problems inherent in current approaches for establishing capitation payment rates, it is important to consider what happens when capitation rates are not set appropriately. The major problem is that inappropriate rates provide a very strong incentive for providers to try to achieve favorable risk selection. Favorable selection occurs when individuals enrolling in capitated health plans have predictable expenses that are lower than the premium charged for them to enroll in those plans (Luft 1978).

HMOs could achieve favorable selection through a number of deliberate actions. They could, for example, locate their facilities in areas known to have low utilization rates; advertise in locations or ways that are most likely to attract healthier individuals; or implement practices that encourage high-risk individuals or those with multiple medical problems to disenroll. Favorable selection will also tend to occur naturally, since individuals who have established ties with physicians, and hence are least likely to enroll in closed-panel capitated plans, are most likely to have a history of medical problems (Anderson et al. 1986b; Luft 1978).

In a situation in which favorable selection occurs, the health care costs of a third-party payer that provides its beneficiaries with a choice between FFS and capitated provider options could increase markedly (Anderson et al. 1986b). In the case of the Medicare program, for example, in which half of the beneficiaries use no covered services in any given year (Anderson and Knickman 1984), the total program cost could increase markedly if a disproportionate share of low-risk individuals enrolled in prepaid plans at a cost to Medicare of 95 percent of the AAPCC. In the process, the providers who achieved favorable selection could realize large profits unrelated to efficiencies in the provision of health care. Any capitated providers unfortunate enough to enroll an adverse selection of beneficiaries, in contrast, would be likely to lose money for reasons unrelated to inefficiencies in their provision of health care.

The second major problem that could occur if capitation premium rates were not established appropriately would be that high-risk individuals might have difficulty gaining access to prepaid care. Access of high-risk individuals to conventional insurance for the FFS sector might also become limited as the price of comprehensive coverage increased in response to depletion of low-risk individuals from the risk pool for such insurance. Limitations on high-risk individuals' access to either prepaid or insured FFS health care might also arise in a situation in which capitation payment rates were set solely by the marketplace (Anderson et al. 1986b).

Summary

During the past fifteen years interest in HMOs in this country has increased sharply, manifested by an increase in nationwide enrollment from

3 million in 1971 to 31 million in 1988. Over the last ten years the proportion of the U.S. population enrolled in HMOs has increased from 3 percent to approximately 13 percent.

This increased interest in HMOs is due primarily to a belief that they provide health care equal in quality to that provided by the FFS sector but at a lower cost. This belief is substantiated by a growing body of evidence. In a detailed review of the literature, for example, Luft found that total annual costs per person were 10–40 percent lower for HMO enrollees than for non-HMO enrollees (Luft 1978, 1981). A recent study by Rand also found that annual expenditures among HMO enrollees were about 25 percent lower than those of individuals cared for in the FFS sector (Manning et al. 1984). In both studies the lower costs among HMO enrollees were attributable to fewer hospital admissions and fewer total hospital days. No evidence has emerged suggesting that the quality of care offered in HMOs is inferior to that offered in the FFS sector.

HMO penetration has not occurred uniformly across the country. Only six states had more than 20 percent of their population enrolled in HMOs in 1988. Certain SMSAs, such as San Francisco and Minneapolis, had more than 39 percent of their population enrolled in HMOs, however. To date, HMOs have been most likely to establish themselves in areas with a population base of at least 1 million and a large number of working individuals concentrated in a few large firms.

The structure of the HMO industry is also changing rapidly. At least three major trends can be discerned. First, among all types of HMOs, IPA model HMOs have experienced the greatest increases in enrollment in the past two years. Second, affiliations among HMOs, in the form of common ownership, management, and marketing arrangements, are becoming more and more common. Third, the proportion of HMOs operating as for-profit entities has increased sharply, from 18 percent in 1982 to 67 percent in 1988. It is unclear as yet what the effect of these changes will be on the future performance of the HMO industry. Because physicians in IPA model HMOs can contract with several HMOs, and because HMO enrollees may constitute only a small proportion of any IPA physician's practice, there is some question whether physician loyalty to the HMO will be as strong in IPA model HMOs and whether IPA model HMOs will cut costs as effectively as other HMO models. The increase in affiliations among HMOs may lead to economies of scale, but it may also signal the increasing need for a large capital base to ensure financial viability. Finally, the increase in for-profit HMOs may herald a change in the philosophy of the HMO industry compared with that of fifteen years ago, a change that could either increase or decrease the health care cost savings society will derive from HMOs in the future.

Projections about the future magnitude of HMO enrollment are a bit speculative, but they suggest that approximately 15–30 percent of the U.S. population will be enrolled in HMOs by 1995. Competition will come from PPO arrangements as well as from traditional insurers in the FFS sector. Future HMO enrollment will be influenced by the strength of societal concerns about health care costs, the extent to which differentials in the cost of care provided by HMOs and FFS providers continue, local attitudes about the desirability of having a private physician and the freedom to choose where and by whom one is given health care, changes in the supply and the attitudes of physicians, and the strengths and form of future government support and regulation.

At least two types of government regulation of HMOs are likely to receive increased attention in the future. The first relates to capital reserve requirements, which appear to decrease the likelihood of HMO financial failures. The second pertains to the need, given the financial incentives implicit in HMOs, to ensure that HMO enrollees receive highquality care.

Finally, the future role of HMOs in the care of Medicare and Medicaid beneficiaries remains unclear. At present only about 3 percent of such beneficiaries are enrolled in HMOs. Given current beliefs about the cost-saving potential of HMOs, state and federal efforts to increase Medicaid and Medicare beneficiary enrollment in HMOs are likely to increase. Medicaid enrollment in HMOs rose 43 percent between December 1985 and December 1986 to a total of 802,750 in 125 plans (Gruber, Shadle, and Polich 1988). Much of this increase is due to mandatory enrollment in several states, such as Wisconsin. Concerns about abridgment of beneficiaries' freedom of choice may limit the number of states that adopt such a strategy. The magnitude of future Medicare beneficiary enrollment in HMOs, in contrast, is likely to depend in largest part on the development of an equitable methodology for determination of capitation premiums.

There are several barriers to enrolling Medicaid beneficiaries in HMOs, especially on a voluntary basis. It is difficult for an HMO to offer additional services as an inducement to enroll in states where the Medicaid benefit package is already expansive. The emphasis in most of the voluntary programs has been on some sort of an eligibility guarantee as an enrollment incentive. Beneficiary turnover also makes it hard to estimate actual costs of providing care. Plans are unlikely to become involved in serving this population unless they believe that the potential for economic loss is remote (Galblum and Trieger 1982).

While the federal government is moving toward an increased enrollment of Medicare and Medicaid beneficiaries in HMOs, clearly there is justifiable concern that HMO activity be adequately monitored. Improving the payment methodology and protecting beneficiaries from the incentives for underutilization mandate that the government continue to be actively involved in regulating HMOs. Beneficiaries must continue to be assured of their right to disenroll and of grievance procedures. Current legislation would require that independent quality assessments occur (Iglehart 1987). It is equally important to monitor the financial viability of organizations serving the Medicare and Medicaid populations.

Future Directions

The experience with HMOs to date is sufficiently promising to warrant their promotion for Medicare and Medicaid beneficiaries and enrollees of employer health benefit programs. This section outlines our recommendations for promoting HMO enrollment while building in safeguards to ensure quality and financial soundness.

Freedom of choice between HMOs and FFS providers. One important safeguard against abuses that can develop within an HMO plan is to guarantee that enrollees have the right to disenroll and select from a wide range of FFS providers. Maintenance of choice between FFS and capitated plans may provide a guarantee against reductions in quality of care, since the availability of an FFS alternative for HMO enrollees would provide a strong incentive for capitated providers to maintain a high standard of care. If, for example, government payment rates to HMO plans became so low that none of the HMO plans could provide adequate care, an FFS option would provide an attractive alternative.

The benefits of maintaining both traditional insurance and HMO options are more important than any cost savings that may occur as a result of restricting freedom of choice to only capitated providers. Medicaid's experience with HMO-only options (see chapter 4) suggests that quality of care can suffer if beneficiaries are restricted to only one option. Thus, public insurance programs, as well as employer health plans covering more than ten employees, should be required to offer both an HMO and an FFS option. Extending this requirement to smaller employers, however, would be impractical.

If HMO and FFS plans differ in total premium cost for comparable benefits, the individual should pay the cost of selecting the higher-cost option. Exceptions to this policy may have to be made for lower-income enrollees; financial contributions for such enrollees could be waived, or they could be asked to contribute only a portion of the cost differential.

Multiple competing HMOs. The benefits of having multiple competing HMOs are the same as those in any industry. Under the proper conditions, competition can produce cost savings and improve quality. Employers with at least ten employees and public programs such as Medicare and Medicaid should be required to offer beneficiaries multiple HMO plans. The number that are actually offered, however, could be restricted to ensure that only those plans that are believed to provide an adequate benefit package and quality of care are offered. Public and private managers thus would be expected to exercise discretion in limiting the number of plans offered.

In addition, all plans should have enrollees who are drawn from a spectrum of payer sources. Specifically, no more than 50 percent of the enrollees in any HMO should consist of Medicaid or Medicare beneficiaries. Any capitated plan whose enrollees are from a single sources, such as Medicaid, is susceptible to manipulation by the funding source and is more likely to provide substandard care.

Minimum benefits package. In order to reduce the possibility of risk selection, a minimum HMO benefit package should be mandated, comparable to that in the employer minimum health benefits plan described in chapter 6. The availability of a minimum benefit package would help consumers compare the benefits being offered by alternative plans.

Open enrollment. HMOs and private health insurance plans should be required to offer an annual open enrollment period. Insurers would be required to issue policies at actuarially fair rates. This would improve access to health insurance, avoid placing HMOs at a serious financial disadvantage relative to insurance plans, and reduce the bad debt load of providers that comes from refusal to cover individuals who are poor health risks.

Information dissemination. For genuine choice among alternatives to occur, information on which to make informed choices must be widely available. One potential solution to reducing the confusion regarding the diversity of coverage, benefits, and cost sharing among alternative plans is to provide enrollees with personal counseling. Counseling services should be made available to all potential enrollees by their employer or union, the government, or whoever is providing the health care coverage.

Preventing risk selection. HMOs have a financial incentive to avoid patients who are poor health risks or who are likely to incur higher health expenditures. HMOs may discourage the enrollment of such individuals, or encourage them to disenroll once they have enrolled. The most effective way to reduce these incentives is to establish an HMO capitation rate that is based on the anticipated medical expenditures of enrollees (Anderson et al. 1986b).

Premium rates. While the expected cost of caring for some enrollees will be greater than that of caring for others, it does not necessarily follow that these higher costs should be borne by these individuals. Rather, the premiums paid on behalf of enrollees by either employers or government payers should be adjusted for the anticipated health expenditures of those enrollees so that sicker enrollees do not themselves have to pay more simply because of their greater health service needs. In other words, although individuals' premiums should be allowed to vary if they elect less efficient plans, they should not vary as a function of the anticipated health status of the enrollee. Private sector and government health insurance benefit packages thus should be structured not only to allow higher payments to providers on behalf of sicker individuals but also to protect sicker individuals from having to pay higher premiums themselves.

Guaranteeing quality care. Monitoring quality of care in HMO plans is especially important because consumers who enroll in them must pay out-ofpocket to see a nonplan physician and because providers practicing in them have a financial incentive to limit the services they provide to their patients. A major debate exists over whether competition or regulation offers better approaches to assurance of high-quality care. Competition will promote high-quality care if patients are able to assess quality. Because measures of quality, especially outcome measures, tend to be extremely crude, publication of comparative statistics would provide a very limited, if not misleading, indication of the quality of care provided in different settings. This difficulty in assessing quality will limit the ability of the competitive process to promote quality. Similarly, a regulatory approach will experience difficulties in ensuring high-quality care if adequate measures of quality are not available. Currently, few process or outcome measures are available to monitor quality in either capitation or FFS plans. As a result, even if highly trained professionals are used, most regulatory solutions will tend to employ structural measures, such as availability of services and numbers of personnel, as indexes of quality.

The government and the medical profession should begin to develop quality measures and to use them to monitor the quality of care in HMOs. The government should set minimum quality standards for federal certification of HMOs and monitor these systems to make sure the standards are met. Only federally certified plans should be made available to Medicare and Medicaid enrollees, and employers should be encouraged to use federal certification as a criterion for offering a plan to employees. Some provisions are also necessary to assure that HMOs are financially sound. Criteria regarding financial soundness should be a part of the federal certification process.

Summary

As the number of HMOs increases it will be necessary to make a number of policy choices. Many of these choices potentially involve tradeoffs between cost containment and access to and quality of care. In reviewing the various alternatives, we recommend the following:

- Require freedom of choice between FFS and HMOs for all Medicare and Medicaid beneficiaries and all employees of firms with more than ten employees
- Require multiple capitated plans to be offered wherever possible and ensure that no more than half of the enrollees in any plan are drawn from a single payer source
- Mandate a minimum benefit package for all plans
- Require all HMOs and insurance plans to offer open enrollment periods
- Require information on the various options to be provided by employers, unions, government, or whoever is providing services
- Adjust HMO capitation payment rates for anticipated health status but do not permit premiums paid by enrollees to vary with health status
- Require federal certification of HMOs based on quality of care and financial soundness criteria

Chapter 8

The Effectiveness of Cost
Containment Efforts in Containing
Health Care Costs, 1950–1987

The public and private sectors have been involved with cost containment efforts for decades. In the 1930s the Commission on the Cost of Medical Care examined the performance of the health sector and made major recommendations to improve efficiency and curb the upward spiral in health care costs. Concern with rising health care costs has been particularly acute for the last two decades. Every administration since that of Lyndon Johnson has issued major reports, mounted programs, or developed legislative proposals to deal with the problem.

This chapter summarizes the major trends in health care costs over the period 1950–87 that have caused this attention and presents the available evidence on the effectiveness of cost containment approaches in restraining rates of increase. The period 1950–87 is important in several respects. The period is marked by major expansion of health insurance coverage, beginning with the growth of employment-based group health insurance in the 1950s and followed by major growth in federal and state government expenditures for health care services in the period 1965–87. It is also characterized by numerous attempts by the federal and state governments and by the private sector to restrain cost increases.

National Health Expenditures

Trends, 1950–1987

National health expenditures rose sharply throughout the period 1950–87. In 1950 the nation spent $12.7 billion on the health sector; by 1987 national health spending had increased to $497 billion (see table 8.1). In other words, in 1950 the nation spent a billion dollars on health every month; by 1987 it spent well over a billion dollars a day. Translated into personal terms, the nation spent $80 per person in 1950; by 1987 that figure was $1,973 (Anderson and Erickson 1987).

Table 8.1. National Health Expenditures, Percentage of Gross National Product, and Annualized Percentage Change, Selected Calendar Years, 1950–1987

| Calendar Year | National Health Expenditures | | |
	Total ($ billions)	Per Capita ($)	As Percentage of GNP
1950	12.7	80	4.4
1955	17.7	101	4.4
1960	26.9	142	5.2
1965	41.9	205	5.9
1970	75.0	349	7.4
1975	132.7	591	8.3
1980	248.1	1,054	9.1
1985	422.6	1,710	10.6
1986	458.2	1,837	10.9
1987	497.0	1,973	11.2
Percentage change (annualized), 1950–87	10.4	9.0	

Sources: Levit et al. 1985; HCFA 1987b.

Throughout this period spending on health outpaced spending in the rest of the economy. Health spending as a percentage of the Gross National Product (GNP) increased steadily from 4.4 percent in 1950 to 11.2 percent in 1987. As more of the nation's income was being spent on health care, relatively less was left over for food, housing, and other nonhealth care goods and services. The annualized rate of increase in health expenditures was 10.4 percent from 1950 to 1987, compared with an annual increase in the GNP of 7.7 percent. In other words, health spending increased about 3 percent per year faster than spending in the rest of the economy.

Real Growth in National Health Expenditures

Trends in the health sector are partially dependent on general trends in the economy. Not surprisingly, during periods of overall price inflation, expenditures in the health sector rise only more rapidly. It is important in any analysis of health care cost increases to look at the pattern of increases that are over and above those that can be attributed to wide inflation.

To evaluate real growth, expenditures over time must be made comparable through the use of constant dollars. Table 8.2 presents trends in national health expenditures deflated by the Consumer Price Index, or CPI (deflating by the Gross National Product implicit price deflator yields similar results). As shown, national health expenditures in constant 1967

Table 8.2. National Health Expenditures in Constant 1967 Dollars, Per Capita, and Annualized Percentage Change, Selected Calendar Years, 1950–1987

	Real National Health Expenditures	
Calendar Year	Amount ($ billions)	Per Capita ($)
1950	17.6	116
1955	22.1	133
1960	30.3	167
1965	44.3	228
1970	64.5	315
1975	82.3	381
1980	100.5	443
1985	131.2	549
1986	139.5	579
1987	146.0	580
Percentage change (annualized), 1950–87	5.9	4.4

Sources: Calculated from Levit et al. 1985; Census 1987b; and HCFA 1987b.
Note: Actual dollar amounts were deflated by the Consumer Price Index (1967 = 100).

dollars increased from $17.6 billion in 1950 to $146 billion in 1987. Per capita expenditures rose from $116 in 1950 to $580 in 1987. The real rate of growth in national health spending averaged 5.9 percent annually over the period.

Trends in National Health Expenditures for Selected Periods

Breaking the trends in national health expenditures down by time periods related to major shifts in health financing policy yields interesting insights. Seven time periods are of particular importance:

- Growth in private health insurance, 1950–65
- Early Medicare and Medicaid, 1966–71
- The Economic Stabilization Program, 1972–74
- The Post–Economic Stabilization Program, 1975–77
- The hospital cost containment bill and the hospital industry Voluntary Effort, 1978–80
- The market era, 1981–83
- The Medicare Prospective Payment System, 1984–87

Most of the cost containment initiatives in these various periods applied only to hospitals. Still, they probably had some effect on total health spending, since hospital services account for about 40 percent of all health

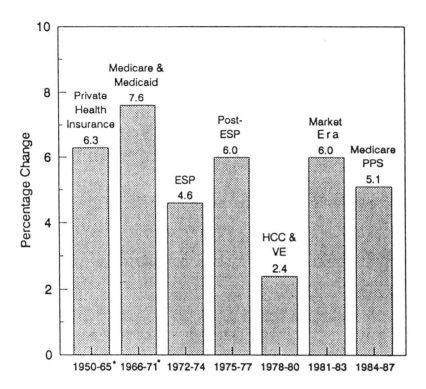

* Annualized

Fig. 8.1. **The Average Annual Rate of Increase in Real National Health Expenditures, 1950–1987**
(*Source:* Calculated from Levit et al. 1985; Census 1987b; and HCFA 1987b.)

outlays. Moreover, it is important to view the health sector as a whole to determine whether initiatives to control hospital costs are offset by increased expenditures for nonhospital services.

Figure 8.1 shows the annual rate of increase in real national health expenditures over the 1950–87 period. Real national health expenditures increased most rapidly during periods of expanding health insurance coverage or following the relaxation of mandatory or voluntary controls on the health care sector. By far the slowest rates of increase in real health care expenditures occurred during periods when mandatory limits were either threatened or imposed. During the Economic Stabilization Program real increases in expenditures averaged 4.6 percent annually. Under the threat of the Carter hospital cost containment bill and the subsequent hospital industry Voluntary Effort response, real increases averaged 2.4

percent. Real rates of increase in health expenditures averaged 5.1 percent during the first three years of the Medicare PPS. By contrast, the highest rates of increase occurred during the periods of expanded public and private insurance coverage and following the Economic Stabilization Program.

The Nation's Health Care Dollar: Where Does It Come From and Where Does It Go?

Health care in the United States is financed by a mix of public and private funds. As shown in figure 8.2, federal, state, and local governments pay for about 40 percent of health expenditures, private health insurance pays for another 31 percent, and the remainder comes directly from patients, philanthropy, and other private sources. Medicare and Medicaid make up the largest share of the public financing and together represent the source of 29 percent of all the health care dollars.

Table 8.3 indicates trends over time in sources of financing personal health care services (which exclude research, construction, and administration). Over the period 1950–87 the private health insurance industry grew from a $1 billion industry to a $154.7 billion industry (HCFA 1987b). In 1950 private health insurance financed 9.1 percent of personal health care expenditures. This number grew steadily between 1950 and the early 1980s, peaking at 31.9 percent in 1982 and dropping slightly to 31 percent in 1987.

State and local government spending on health care as a share of all health expenditures has been relatively stable over the 1950–87 period, averaging between 9 percent and 13 percent. The share paid by state and local government hit a high of 12.7 percent in 1975 and declined gradually to 9.3 percent in 1987. Federal government health expenditures rose from 10.4 percent of the health care bill in 1950 to 29.3 percent in 1987. The federal share took a major shift upward with passage of Medicare and Medicaid in 1965, rising again in 1972 with the expansion of Medicare coverage to the disabled. Federal expenditures have since continued to grow gradually as the population ages.

The share of personal health expenditures paid directly by patients out-of-pocket declined from 65.5 percent in 1950 to 27.1 percent in 1982 and crept up slightly to 29.1 percent of all expenditures in 1987. Cutbacks in Medicare, Medicaid, and private health insurance plans appear to be shifting more of the cost of health care directly onto patients. With the rapid rise in health expenditures, even a small increase in share can have a substantial dollar impact. In 1980 Americans paid $268 per person directly out-of-pocket for personal health care services; in 1987 this had increased to $508 (HCFA 1987b).

Where it came from

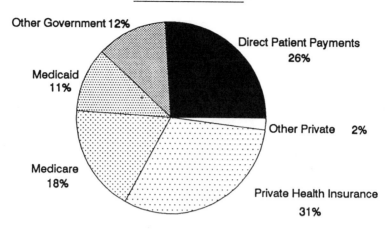

Other Government 12%

Direct Patient Payments
26%

Medicaid
11%

Other Private   2%

Medicare
18%

Private Health Insurance
31%

And where it went

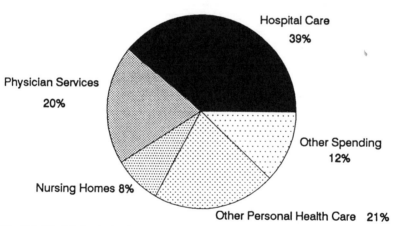

Hospital Care
39%

Physician Services
20%

Other Spending
12%

Nursing Homes 8%

Other Personal Health Care   21%

Fig. 8.2. **The Nation's Health Care Dollar, 1987**
(*Source:* HCFA 1987b.)

Hospital care was the largest and one of the fastest growing services over the 1950–87 period. Spending for hospital care as a percentage of all personal health care spending increased from 35.8 percent in 1950 to 44 percent in 1987 (HCFA 1987b). In the period 1984–87 hospital expenditure rates of increase slowed to about 7 percent. This was slower than the historical rate of growth and much slower than that of other health care providers.

Table 8.3. Percentage Distribution of Personal Health Care Expenditures by Source of Funds, Selected Calendar Years, 1950–1987

| Calendar Year | Total | Direct Patient Payments | Third Parties | | | | Government | |
			Total Third Parties	Private Health Insurance	Other Private Funds	Total Government	Federal	State and Local
1950	100.0	65.5	34.5	9.1	2.9	22.4	10.4	12.0
1955	100.0	58.1	41.9	16.1	2.8	23.0	10.5	12.5
1960	100.0	54.9	45.1	21.1	2.3	21.8	9.3	12.5
1965	100.0	51.6	48.4	24.2	2.2	22.0	10.1	11.9
1967	100.0	42.6	57.4	21.6	1.9	33.9	21.3	12.6
1970	100.0	40.5	59.5	23.4	1.7	34.3	22.2	12.1
1975	100.0	32.5	67.5	26.7	1.3	39.5	26.8	12.7
1980	100.0	28.7	71.3	30.7	1.2	39.4	28.4	10.9
1985	100.0	28.4	71.6	30.4	1.2	40.0	30.3	9.6
1986	100.0	28.7	71.3	30.4	1.2	39.6	30.2	9.4
1987	100.0	29.1	70.9	31.1	1.2	38.6	29.3	9.3

Sources: Levit et al. 1985; HCFA 1987b.

Table 8.4. Community Hospital Expenses per Stay and per Patient Day, Selected Calendar Years, 1950–1987

Calendar Year	Total ($ billions)	Per Hospital Stay[a] ($)	Per Patient Day[a] ($)
1950	2.1	127	16
1955	3.4	180	23
1960	5.6	244	32
1965	9.1	316	41
1970	19.6	605	74
1975	39.1	1,024	133
1980	76.8	1,851	245
1985	130.5	3,245	460
1986	140.6	3,532	501
1987	152.6	3,850	539
Percentage increase (annualized), 1950–87	12.3%	9.7%	10.0%

Source: Calculated from data in AHA 1988.

Note: Community hospital expenses include all nonfederal, short-term general, and other special hospital expenses.

[a]Adjusted for outpatient visits for the years 1965–87.

Physician services are the second largest item in personal health care spending, accounting for 23 percent of expenditures in 1987, down slightly from 24.8 percent in 1950. Nursing home care spending has increased rapidly, especially since Medicaid was introduced in 1965. In 1950 nursing home expenses represented only 1.8 percent of all personal health care spending; this had increased to 5.9 percent in 1965 and rose to 9.5 percent in 1987. The remaining 23.5 percent of personal care spending in 1987 came from drugs, dental care, eyeglasses and appliances, other professional services, and other personal health care services.

Hospital Care

Trends in Community Hospital Expenses, 1950–1987

As the largest and one of the most rapidly growing components of personal health care spending, hospital care is especially significant. As shown in table 8.4, community hospital spending (including all nonfederal short-term general and other special hospitals) increased from $2.1 billion in 1950 to $152.6 billion in 1987. For each patient admitted to a hospital, the average cost rose from $127 in 1950 to $3,850 in 1987 (data are based on annual surveys of all hospitals conducted by the AHA). A day in the hospital cost $16 in 1950; in 1987 it cost $539. Expressed as an

Table 8.5. **Real Community Hospital Expenses per Stay and per Patient Day in Constant 1967 Dollars, Selected Calendar Years, 1950–1987**

Calendar Year	Total ($ billions)	Per Hospital Stay[a] ($)	Per Patient Day[a] ($)
1950	2.9	176	22
1955	4.2	224	29
1960	6.3	275	36
1965	9.6	335	43
1970	16.8	520	64
1975	24.2	639	83
1980	31.1	750	99
1985	40.5	1,007	143
1986	42.8	1,076	152
1987	44.8	1,131	158
Percentage increase (annualized), 1950–87	7.7%	5.2%	5.5%

Source: Calculated from AHA 1988.

Note: Community hospital expenses includes all nonfederal, short-term general, and other special hospital expenses deflated by the Consumer Price Index (1967 = 100).

[a]Adjusted for outpatient visits for the years 1965–87.

annualized percentage increase, total community hospital expenses increased 12.3 percent from 1950 to 1987, while expenses per hospital stay increased by 9.7 percent, and expenses per patient day increased by 10 percent.

Real Increases in Hospital Expenses

Some portion of the increase in hospital expenditures can be traced to inflation in the economy as a whole. To understand trends in the hospital sector, it is important to focus on hospital expenses deflated by general economic inflation. Table 8.5 presents trends over the 1950–87 period, with community hospital expenses deflated by the CPI. In constant 1967 dollars, hospital expenses increased from $2.9 billion in 1950 to $44.8 billion in 1987. For each patient admitted to a hospital, the average real cost rose from $176 in 1950 to $1,131 in 1987. A day in the hospital cost $22 in constant 1967 dollars in 1950; in 1987 it cost $158. Expressed as an annualized percentage increase, real community hospital expenses increased by 7.7 percent from 1950 to 1987, while expenses per hospital stay increased by 5.2 percent, and expenses per patient day increased by 5.5 percent.

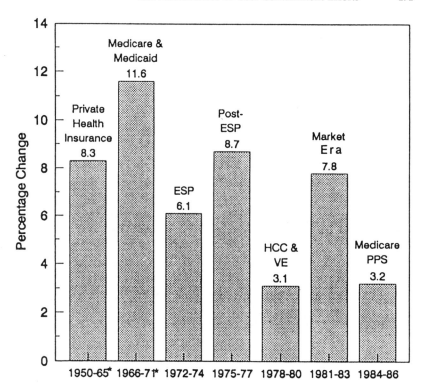

* Annualized

Fig. 8.3. **The Average Annual Rate of Increase in Real Community Hospital Expenses, 1950–1986**
(*Source:* Calculated from AHA and Census data, 1950–86.)

Trends in Real Hospital Expenses for Selected Periods

Figure 8.3 indicates that hospital spending is particularly sensitive to government intervention. The lowest rates of increase in real hospital spending occurred during periods of mandatory limits on hospital payments or when there was a threat of such mandatory limits. During the Economic Stabilization Program real increases in hospital expenditures averaged 6.1 percent annually; during the first three years of the Medicare PPS, increases in hospital spending averaged 3.2 percent annually; and under the threat of the Carter hospital cost containment bill with the hospital industry Voluntary Effort response, real increases averaged 3.1 percent. By contrast, the highest rates of increase were following the Economic Stabilization Program (8.7 percent) and following the defeat of the Carter hospital cost containment bill (7.8 percent).

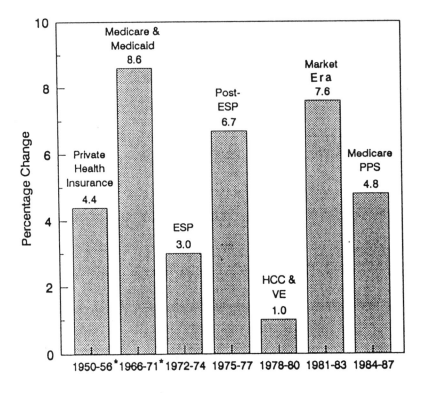

* Annualized
Fig. 8.4. **The Average Annual Rate of Increase in Real Community Hospital Expenses, per Hospital Stay, 1950–1986**
(*Source:* Calculated from AHA and Census data, 1950–86.)

Trends in real hospital expenses per hospital admission and per day of hospital care are similar with one notable exception: in 1984–86, under implementation of the Medicare PPS, real hospital costs per stay increased slowly (4.8 percent), but hospital costs per patient day continued to increase substantially in real terms (7.0 percent) (see figs. 8.4 and 8.5). This indicates that much of the abatement in total hospital expenses in the last period was a reflection of declining admissions and lengths of hospital stay, not a reduction in the rate of increase in the cost of a day of care.

Throughout the 1950–86 period real hospital costs per day of care increased at an annualized rate of 7.0 percent. This increase is sometimes referred to as the "intensity" factor. It reflects increases in hospital costs that cannot be explained by general economic inflation, increases in the population, or more days of hospital care per capita. It represents the

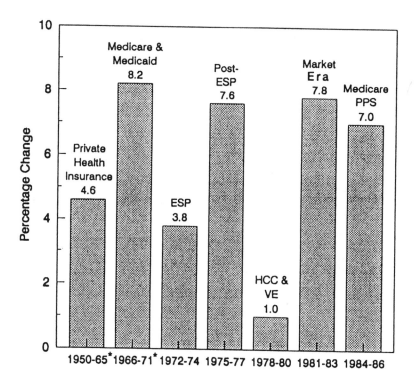

* Annualized

Fig. 8.5. **The Average Annual Rate of Increase in Real Community Hospital Expenses, per Patient Day, 1950–1986**
(*Source:* Calculated from AHA and Census data, 1950–86.)

increasing complexity of hospital care, the greater use of specialized personnel or capital equipment to provide a given day of care, and changes in technology, quality, or style of hospital care.

Greater intensity of hospital care is described in terms of more laboratory and radiological tests, such as CT scans or magnetic resonance imaging; more specialized services, such as burn units or intensive cardiac or neonatal care units; more complex surgery, such as transplantation; and better patient amenities. Increases in hospital costs that are not explained by inflation are of particular concern to analysts and policy officials. Service intensity can only be justified if greater intensity has concomitant benefits in terms of improved patient care or health outcomes. In fact, in most industries increasing productivity and efficiency would require fewer resources over time to provide a given level of output. This has not been true for hospitals.

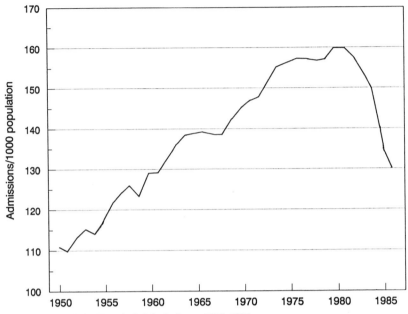

Fig. 8.6. **Trends in Hospital Admissions, 1950–1986**
(*Source:* Calculated from AHA and Census data, 1950–86.)

Any improvements in efficiency and productivity that have occurred in the hospital sector have been overshadowed by ever rising resource requirements to provide a different form of care (Davis et al. 1985). Policy efforts to contain hospital costs, therefore, have focused on measures to reduce the intensity factor rather than on the prices hospitals charge for specific services (such as laboratory tests) or on hospital profits.

Utilization of Hospital Services

Trends in hospital utilization are also important in understanding total hospital spending over the 1950–87 period (see fig. 8.6). Admissions to hospitals generally increased faster than would be explained on the basis of population growth or the aging of the population. Hospital admissions per capita increased at a relatively steady rate up until 1980. Since the early 1980s, however, hospital admissions per capita have begun to decline, especially during 1982–87.

Patterns of the average numbers of days that patients stayed in the hospital during this period are also interesting. The length of hospital stay declined from 1950 to the early 1960s (see fig. 8.7). The effects of penicillin and changing medical practice (e.g., having patients walk

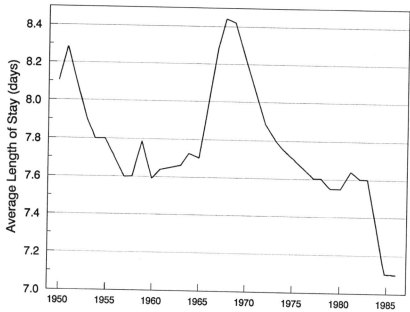

Fig. 8.7. **Trends in Average Length of Stay, 1950–1986**
(*Source:* Calculated from AHA and Census data, 1950–86.)

sooner after surgery and after delivering a baby) are generally held responsible for the reduced length of stay over the 1950s. The average length of stay jumped precipitously in the late 1960s. This is widely attributed to the introduction of the Medicare program. Patients over age sixty-five displaced younger patients, leading to a longer average stay. The average length of stay, however, turned down again sharply in the early 1970s and flattened out in the late 1970s. Lengths of stay have taken another sharp decline since 1983.

The combined effect of changes in admissions per 1,000 population and average length of hospital stay is reflected in the trends of total hospital patient days per 1,000 population. As shown in figure 8.8, patient days per 1,000 population rose steadily through the 1950s, went through a rather marked increase in the 1960s, increased somewhat erratically over the 1970s, and moved sharply downward in the early 1980s.

The early 1980s are such a major departure from the earlier historical period that more detailed examination is in order. As shown in figure 8.9, the National Hospital Panel Survey shows that admissions for patients under age sixty-five have been the major source of decline during the early 1980s, with relatively stable admission rates for patients age

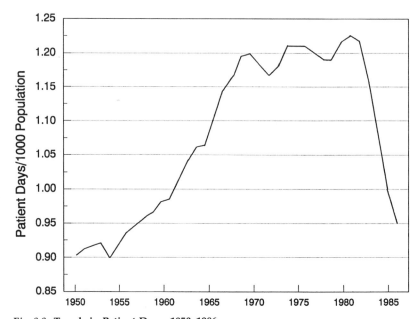

Fig. 8.8. **Trends in Patient Days, 1950–1986**
(*Source:* Calculated from AHA and Census data, 1950–86.)

sixty-five and over. However, though their admission rates have been stable, the average length of stay for patients age sixty-five and over has declined quite sharply during this period. Nonelderly patients have experienced only moderate declines in length of stay (HCFA 1987b).

The decline in utilization of hospital services by both the elderly and the nonelderly is largely responsible for the abatement in real hospital cost increases in the early 1980s. The slowdown in use of hospital services in the early 1980s may be explained by a number of factors. First, the adoption of the Medicare PPS for hospitals offered a strong incentive to hospitals to shorten the lengths of stay of the Medicare population. There is arguably a spillover effect onto the non-Medicare population: to the extent that physicians are changing their practice patterns in response to the incentives inherent in a Medicare patient, their treatment of other patients may also be expected to change.

A second factor plausibly responsible for the decline in utilization has been the recent growth in the number of HMO enrollees. HMOs and other capitated financing arrangements contain much stronger disincentives to admit patients, and even when they are admitted, there are stronger incentives (in comparison with those in the FFS system) to keep

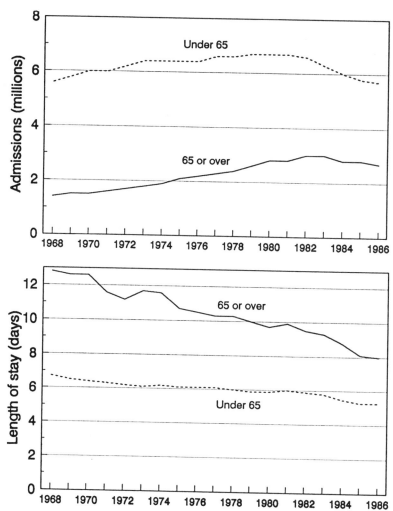

Fig. 8.9. The Number of Community Hospital Admissions and Length of Stay for Populations under Age 65 and Age 65 or Over, Calendar Years 1968–1986 (*Source:* HCFA 1987b.)

them in the hospital for relatively shorter periods. As of 1987, HMOs attracted more than 30 million enrollees nationally, and their membership growth suggests that they will soon be more than a regional phenomenon (GHAA 1988b). Recent studies conclude that HMOs effect decreases in hospital admissions of up to 40 percent (Manning et al. 1984). PPOs, while retaining the characteristic of reimbursement on an FFS basis, may have also contributed to declines in admissions and length of stay. In return for guaranteed volumes of patients at discounted prices, such contracting providers usually must agree to a stringent utilization review process.

Third, the proliferation of treatment settings that can serve as substitutes for inpatient hospitalization—mainly those delivering ambulatory or outpatient care but also home health and other institutional settings—may have diverted patients away from inpatient settings or siphoned them out of hospitals earlier. Freestanding emergency and surgical centers, in delivering single-day treatments, may force hospitals to compete for similar patients, resulting in a lowering of the hospital's average length of stay.

Fourth, the increasing burden of cost sharing that insured patients have been asked to shoulder has probably also contributed to the decline in admissions. Private and public insurers have raised deductible and coinsurance levels, and employers have offered financial incentives to employees selecting less comprehensive plans or those with higher out-of-pocket requirements (Newhouse et al. 1981).

Fifth, greater emphasis on utilization review, both prior and subsequent to a hospital stay, on the part of hospitals, insurers, and employers may also be responsible for the declines in admissions and length of stay. Many insurance plans or selective contracting arrangements now require preadmission testing, second-opinion surgery, or postdischarge planning. Similarly, many businesses, as the "ultimate" payers of hospitalization insurance premiums, have stepped up their claims review efforts in order to detect and reduce unnecessary admissions and days of care.

Sixth, the declines in admissions and lengths of stay may also be due in part to changes in clinical practice patterns and changes resulting from the introduction of new technologies. Greater impetus for a reevaluation of traditional practice styles is being provided by the incentives inherent in PPS. Furthermore, detecting and monitoring of practice patterns has become easier with the advances in hospital management information systems. Likewise, some new technologies and devices have been responsible for shortening lengths of stay. The use of lasers, for example, has been successful in reducing recovery periods for certain types of eye surgery.

Hospital Employment and Labor Costs

Total hospital employment increased steadily from 0.5 million full-time equivalents (FTEs) in 1950 to a peak of 3.1 million in 1982, an annualized rate of growth of 5.9 percent. During the period 1983–86, however, hospital FTEs did not continue to increase but remained fairly constant at about 3 million. The number of full-time employees per patient census increased from 1.8 in 1950 to 3.9 in 1986.

Average hospital employee salaries increased more slowly during the Economic Stabilization Program and while the Carter administration's hospital cost containment proposal was under consideration. In the early 1980s a disproportionate inflation in hospital employee salaries resumed.

Medical Care Prices

Trends in prices charged for individual health care services have generally been of less interest than total expenditures. In large part this is because patients are concerned about the total payment for care, not what he or she is billed for any one service. It is the aggregate of expenditures that affects health insurance premiums and taxes required to support Medicare, Medicaid, and other publicly financed health care services. Nevertheless, comparing health care prices with prices in the general economy provides some insight into the relationship between health care prices and overall health care expenditures. A closer look suggests that unconstrained health care price increases are part of the explanation behind rising health expenditures.

Table 8.6 presents data on annual rates of increase in the CPI for the years 1965–87. Overall economic inflation was strongest in the early Vietnam period (1968–71); it dropped to low rates under President Nixon's Economic Stabilization Program only to be immediately undone by OPEC price increases in 1974. General economic inflation hit double-digit levels in 1974 and again—with another round of OPEC price increases—in 1979.

Subtracting price increases in the overall CPI from price increases in medical care and physicians' services indexes shows a pattern somewhat similar to that observed for real changes in national health expenditures and community hospital expenses. In the years following the introduction of Medicare and Medicaid, the rates of increase in health care prices were high relative to the economywide trend. From 1965 to 1971 medical care prices increased 1.8 percent faster than the CPI, and physicians' services prices increased 2.3 percent faster than the CPI. Under the Economic Stabilization Program in 1972–74 the health sector increased at a slower rate than other sectors. Following the lifting of ESP controls, medical care prices shot up again. Average annual increases over the period 1975–77 were 3.2 percent for all medical care and 3.9 percent for physicians' services. Medical care and physicians' services prices increased at a slower rate than general inflation in the Carter period, from 1978 to 1980, and have been several percentage points above general inflation since 1981.

Table 8.6. Average Percentage Change in the Consumer Price Index, 1965–1987

Year	CPI, All Items	Medical Care Less Increase in CPI	Physician Services Less Increase in CPI
1965	1.7	0.8	1.9
1966	2.9	1.5	2.9
1967	2.9	4.2	4.2
1968	4.2	1.9	1.4
1969	5.4	1.5	1.5
1970	5.9	0.4	1.6
1971	4.3	2.2	2.6
1972	3.3	−0.1	−0.2
1973	6.2	−2.3	−2.9
1974	11.0	−1.7	−1.8
1975	9.1	2.9	3.2
1976	5.8	3.7	5.6
1977	6.5	3.1	2.8
1978	7.7	0.7	0.6
1979	11.3	2.0	2.1
1980	13.5	−2.6	−2.9
1981	10.4	0.4	0.6
1982	6.1	5.5	3.3
1983	3.2	5.5	4.5
1984	4.3	1.9	2.7
1985	3.6	2.6	2.2
1986	1.9	5.6	5.3
1987	3.7	2.8	3.5
Average, 1965–87	6.3	1.9	1.9

Sources: Calculated from HCFA 1987b; Census 1987b; U.S. Department of Labor, Bureau of Labor Statistics 1988.
Note: In adjusting for the CPI, the CPI for all urban consumers was used.

Summary

The health sector has consumed an increasing share of the nation's economic resources over time. The financial burdens of paying for health care services have created concerns for patients, employers, and others paying private health insurance premiums, as well as for taxpayers supporting Medicare and Medicaid.

Despite the central message that health care costs are always increasing, there was a distinct pattern in periods that contained proposed or implemented interventions to control rising health care costs. The Economic Stabilization Program was the first major period to experience a slowdown in health cost increases. During this period prices of health services rose less rapidly than the prices of other goods and services, and community hospital expenses per day of hospital care provided rose at an unusually slow rate. The removal of the ESP controls, however, led to a very rapid acceleration in health care spending.

The legislative proposal to place mandatory limits on hospital revenues proposed by the Carter administration in 1977 and considered by Congress until its defeat in the fall of 1979 coincided with a marked slowdown in community hospital expense increases. The hospital industry then mounted a Voluntary Effort, arguing that hospital costs could be held in check without federal legislation. Hospital costs per patient day in 1978 and 1979 did not increase at all in real terms. This period was remarkably successful in containing costs in the hospital sector—a largely unnoticed and unheralded achievement.

The removal of any threat of federal controls with the defeat of the legislation in the fall of 1979 led to an immediate resumption in rising health care costs. Despite the rhetoric surrounding the Reagan administration's emphasis on stimulating a competitive health care marketplace to contain costs, the early 1980s were characterized by large increases in health care expenditures. From 1981 to 1983 community hospital expenses increased at an annual rate of 7.8 percent in real terms.

The congressional action that set hospital payment limits under Medicare on a per-patient basis as of 1982 caused rates of increase in real hospital spending to moderate. The average length of stay in hospitals shortened dramatically, particularly for patients age sixty-five and over. Hospital admissions of both elderly and nonelderly patients declined. Thus, hospital cost abatement was very much utilization-driven. Real hospital costs per day, however, continued to increase markedly.

Slowdowns in real hospital spending did not find a counterpart in other services. Fees for physician services continued to increase much faster than the CPI. Spending on nonhospital services caused real national health expenditures to continue to increase at historically high rates. The slowdown in hospital spending that occurred during the 1984–87 period resulted from a reduction in utilization of hospital services, specifically a reduction in hospital admissions and a shortening of hospital stays.

Chapter 9

**The Impact of Cost Containment
on Hospital Care to the Poor and
Uninsured**

As public and private payers seek to limit hospital payments, where the
poor obtain their hospital care and how that care is financed have emerged
as major policy issues. The fact that the number of Americans without
insurance coverage is growing raises concerns with regard to health status
and financial barriers to care. It also raises concerns about the fiscal health
of the hospitals that carry the heaviest burden of care for the uninsured.
Cost controls that limit the ability of hospitals to finance indigent care
from other revenue sources potentially affect both access to hospital services for the uninsured and the fiscal viability of hospitals that treat them.
A hospital's payment for care delivered is currently derived from multiple
sources: Medicare pays for the elderly and some disabled, Medicaid covers some of the poor, and Blue Cross and commercial insurers cover most
of the working population. Although the level of payment differs among
these sources, hospitals are assured at least some payment for care rendered to individuals insured under these programs.

The problem of uncompensated care arises because not all individuals
receiving care from hospitals are insured against the cost of that care and
many are poor and unable to pay their medical bills. According to unpublished data from the 1987 Current Population Survey, in 1986 over
37 million Americans had no health insurance coverage from either public
or private programs. The hospitals that cared for the uninsured were
uncompensated for many of the services rendered and had to try to
recoup some of their losses from payments from patients with private
insurance.

This chapter examines hospital care to the poor and the uninsured in
order to assess the impact of cost containment on access to care for the
indigent. The first section reviews recent studies of hospital care to the
uninsured and the role of ownership and academic teaching status on
hospital service to the uninsured. The second section analyzes the dis-

tribution of hospital care to the poor and the uninsured and describes the characteristics of hospitals that care for a high proportion of such patients. The third section assesses the impact of recent cost containment initiatives and limitations on Medicaid hospital coverage on hospital admissions for the poor from 1980 to 1985. The fourth section discusses the policy implications of the distribution of care of the poor and the uninsured among hospitals; and the final section discusses options to assist hospitals caring for the poor.

Previous Research on Hospitals Serving the Poor and the Uninsured

Hospital care for the poor and the uninsured is not distributed evenly among types of hospitals. The major work on hospital care of the indigent has been undertaken collaboratively by Feder, Hadley, and Mullner (1984a, 1984b) using special surveys of hospitals conducted by the AHA in 1980 and 1982 to obtain information on care to the poor and hospitals' financial status. Uncompensated hospital care has also been studied by Sloan, Valvona, and Mullner (1986) using the AHA annual surveys for 1978–82 and the 1981 National Hospital Discharge Survey. Findings from both studies clearly demonstrate that there are significant differences among hospitals in the amount of care they provide to the poor and the uninsured and in the economic consequences of cutbacks in support of care to this population.

Feder, Hadley, and Mullner (1984b) found that in 1980 fewer than 9 percent of the nation's hospitals accounted for 40 percent of all care to the poor on Medicaid and the uninsured. Almost half of these hospitals were in the nation's one hundred largest cities. These hospitals provided a larger share of their care to the poor and treated substantially fewer private-pay patients than other hospitals. Because these hospitals had a smaller share of private patients, they had a smaller revenue base to offset their uncompensated care burden. As a result, one-third of these hospitals, accounting for 15 percent of all care to the poor, ran deficits in 1980. The study concluded that the hospitals' financial situation was due to insufficient revenues and not inefficiency or underuse.

Between 1980 and 1982 the economic recession resulted in substantial increases in the numbers of uninsured and unemployed Americans, as well as in growth in the population in poverty. These economic trends placed increased pressure on hospitals to provide charity care for those with insurance, but the expansion of charity care during the recession did not match the substantial increases in the uninsured population. Between 1980 and 1982 the amount of free care provided by hospitals increased by 3.8 percent, while the number of people who were both poor and inadequately insured increased by almost 21 percent (Feder, Hadley, and Mullner 1984a).

Most hospitals provided only small amounts of free care and did not increase free care in response to increased poverty or uninsurance in their service area. Public hospitals in large cities did increase care, but their expansion was not enough to satisfy the increased demand. In areas where Medicaid enrollment expanded between 1980 and 1982, private hospitals provided more care to the poor, but some of this care was just a shift from public hospitals. Hospitals' proportional effort in providing free care expanded the most when poverty rates increased and Medicaid was expanded to cover additional poor. In general, hospitals did not change their efforts in caring for the poor between 1980 and 1982; thus the distribution of care between public and private hospitals remained relatively unchanged. The failure to expand charity services to meet growing demand meant that some of the poor inevitably fell through the cracks in our health care system.

In recent years many hospitals have attempted to restrict the proportion of nonpaying patients and increase the private pay population (Sloan, Valvona, and Mullner 1986). In most cases, hospitals have not set explicit limits but instead have taken more subtle actions that serve to reduce indigent care levels. This trend is evidenced by the closure of outpatient departments, the construction of outpatient office buildings that are separate from the hospital, reductions in the size of the outpatient department, limits on hospital admissions, and growing pressure on the counties to serve the no-pay population. These actions increasingly limit access to hospitals for the poor and the near-poor (Hanft 1982).

There are increasing reports of uninsured patients being turned away from private hospitals to public hospitals because they are unable to pay (Relman 1985; Wrenn 1985). A California study of patient transfers from fourteen private hospitals to a public facility found that the transferred patients were predominantly young, male, and uninsured and, in some cases, at risk of adverse medical effects from the transfer (Himmelstein et al. 1984). Another study found that nearly 90 percent of the patients transferred from local hospitals to Cook County Hospital, the public hospital in Chicago, had been transferred because they lacked medical insurance; and at the time of transfer one-quarter of the patients were in unstable condition (Schiff et al. 1986).

A high volume of care to indigent patients is closely associated with financial stress for the institution serving the indigent patients. The financial burden of indigent care, like indigent care itself, is not evenly distributed. In 1982 metropolitan hospitals with more than four hundred beds and major teaching programs had uncompensated care burdens of

18.4 percent of gross revenues, compared with levels of less than 4 percent in small, nonteaching hospitals (Sloan, Valvona, and Mullner 1986).

Feder, Hadley, and Mullner (1984b) found that hospitals with a high level of care to the poor were two times as likely to be fiscally stressed year after year as those with a lower level of care. They noted that high proportions of care to indigents and fiscal stress were largely an urban phenomenon: half of the providers with the highest proportion of indigent care were located in the nation's one hundred largest cities. Stressed hospitals obtained more of their revenue from either cost-based or regulated sources of payment and relatively less of their revenue from charge-based commercially insured patients than hospitals with a better fiscal situation. Fiscal stress appears to occur when hospitals lack a sufficient base of surplus-generating patients.

Related research by Hadley and Feder (1985) looked at hospital markup patterns from 1980 to 1982 to determine whether hospitals do in fact shift costs. They found that commercial insurers pay the highest markups but that the capacity to shift costs has limits, and individual hospitals cannot expect to boost markups to commercially insured patients to offset revenue declines fully. Therefore, even with a large private insurance base, hospitals with a heavy uncompensated care burden could face fiscal stress.

Teaching Hospitals and Care for the Poor

Teaching hospitals are a major provider of care to the poor on Medicaid and the uninsured. Sloan, Valvona, and Mullner (1986) found that teaching hospitals had a higher combined charity care and bad debt share than nonteaching hospitals. Feder, Hadley, and Mullner (1984b) found that among the providers with the highest proportion of care to the poor, 10 percent were privately owned teaching hospitals and 13.5 percent were publicly owned teaching hospitals.

Together, public and private teaching hospitals provide 43 percent of all hospital care but 53 percent of all uncompensated care (Commonwealth Fund Task Force 1985). Public hospitals operated by state and local government carry the heaviest load. Public teaching hospitals provide 11 percent of all hospital care in the United States but 31 percent of all uncompensated care. Analyzing AHA revenue data from 1982, Swartz, Newhouse, and Williams (1985) concluded that municipal hospitals with major teaching programs are less financially stable than their nonmunicipal counterparts. They found that hospitals most closely connected with medical schools carried the heaviest burdens and that small teaching hospitals did not differ significantly from other community hospitals.

Assessing the likely impact of cuts in Medicaid hospital spending, Swartz, Newhouse, and Williams concluded that Medicaid constraints did not appear likely to be more serious for teaching facilities than for nonteaching facilities. Of the 307 voluntary hospitals that are teaching hospitals, only 25 (8 percent) are dependent on Medicaid for more than 20 percent of their revenue. Since Medicaid revenues of nonmunicipal teaching hospitals are only 1–4 percent higher than those of nonteaching hospitals, a 20 percent cut in Medicaid would reduce the incomes of teaching hospitals by only 1 percent or less relative to those of their nonteaching competitors (Swartz, Newhouse, and Williams 1985).

Although teaching hospitals are not critically dependent on Medicaid funds, they do receive a disproportionate share of Medicaid hospital payments. In 1978 nearly 70 percent of Medicaid hospital payments went to teaching hospitals, with revenues from Medicaid being most important to public teaching hospitals (Hadley 1983). Teaching hospitals are an important source of care for the poor with Medicaid insurance in part because of the dearth of community physicians who are willing to care for Medicaid patients and admit them to community hospitals. Since many Medicaid patients do not have a private physician, they use the outpatient clinics of teaching hospitals for primary care and are often hospitalized in the teaching hospital attached to the clinic (Sloan and Becker 1984).

Hospital Ownership and Care to the Poor

Public hospitals serve as a major source of care to the poor, especially those without insurance. In 1980 public hospitals provided 22 percent of all U.S. hospital care but 40 percent of all free care (Feder, Hadley, and Mullner 1984b). The large urban public hospitals in the one hundred largest cities carried the heaviest burden, providing 5.5 percent of total care but 20.5 percent of all free care.

Not all public hospitals operate under the same indigent care imperatives. In many rural counties the public hospital is the only community hospital and appears to function more like a voluntary hospital than one under public ownership. Among publicly operated institutions the primary burden for indigent care is borne by seven hundred to eight hundred hospitals located predominately in large cities. These hospitals train 20 percent of the nation's medical and dental residents, operate 42 percent of all burn units, and provide 25 percent of all neonatal intensive care services (R. Brown 1983).

The feasibility of supporting and providing care through public hospitals has come into question with the increasingly competitive nature of the health care system. Many public hospitals have been closed in recent years, and others have been sold or leased to for-profit chains and management companies (R. Brown 1983; Rundal and Limbert 1984). Private ownership and management is viewed as more efficient than the public model, but business incentives are often at odds with the public mandate to be a provider of last resort. This shift to private ownership raises concerns about the continued availability of public hospitals for the poor and especially about the future of the large urban public hospitals with the highest proportion of indigent care (Goff 1980).

Most of the literature on proprietary hospitals and their care to the poor and uninsured is anecdotal or descriptive rather than analytic (Gray 1983; IOM 1986). The mix of patients by payment source is a controversial issue with regard to proprietary hospitals. The proprietary hospitals say that their profits stem from efficiency and that they do their fair share of indigent care, but nonprofit rivals say that the for-profit chains cream the market and neglect the poor (Ermann and Gabel 1984; Sloan and Vraciu 1983).

Creaming refers to practices where the hospital seeks to accept only full-pay patients or elects to deliver only those services that are profitable. This can be accomplished in a variety of ways, including recruiting medical staff who practice in affluent communities, locating in areas less likely to be populated by the uninsured, and refusing outright to give care to the uninsured (Pattison and Katz 1983).

The evidence on the behavior of proprietary hospitals is mixed and inconclusive. Several recent studies have compared proprietary hospitals with nonprofit facilities in terms of costs and concluded that proprietary facilities are more costly for charge payers and have higher costs for ancillary and administrative services (Lewin, Derzon, and Marguilies 1981; Renn et al. 1985). On the issue of creaming, for-profit hospitals appear to treat fewer patients in categories that account for large proportions of uncompensated care, most notably obstetrical services and neonatal intensive care, and tend to locate in areas where there are high levels of privately insured patients (Mullner and Hadley 1984; Renn et al. 1985; Sloan and Vraciu 1983).

Some studies using hospital revenue data have shown that the proportion of care to the uninsured does not appear to differ significantly between forprofit hospitals and voluntary hospitals. Sloan, Valvona, and Mullner (1986) found that proprietary hospitals and private voluntary nonteaching hospitals in similar locations devoted roughly the same percentage of their gross revenue to uncompensated care. In another study of hospitals in Florida, Sloan and Vraciu (1983) found that proprietary hospitals and nonprofit nonteaching hospitals were identical in terms of percentage of patient days for Medicare and Medicaid patients, dollar value of charity care, and bad debt adjustments to revenue.

Locational factors need to be examined further to determine whether the low level of uncompensated care in proprietary hospitals results from admissions policies or a decision to locate in a nonpoverty area. Ermann and Gabel's review (1984) of the available evidence indicates that although multihospital systems and for-profit facilities treat small percentages of Medicaid and uninsured patients, they treat proportionately the same number as nonprofit, independent hospitals in similar market areas. They concluded that if for-profit hospitals cream, they appear to do so by locational choice, not admission discrimination.

Other research studies address the types of patients seen in for-profit hospitals and case mix differences between for-profit and other hospitals. Using discharge data from the Hospital Cost and Utilization Project of the National Center for Health Services Research, Farley (1985) looked at distributions across staged disease categories in public and for-profit hospitals compared with voluntary hospitals. He found that in general for-profit hospitals treat less seriously ill patients than do voluntary or public hospitals and that the differences were most pronounced for the poor on Medicaid and the uninsured.

Summary

The studies undertaken to date demonstrate the importance of examining changes in access to hospital services for the poor and the uninsured. The number of uninsured Americans is growing, but hospitals' willingness to provide charity care does not appear to have expanded to meet the growing demand. Those hospitals that treat the highest proportion of indigent patients appear to have greater financial stress than the institutions that carry a lighter indigent care load (Mulstein 1984).

Cost containment policies are likely to impose additional constraints on the facilities caring for the poor. Controls on government spending for health care have intensified in the 1980s. Medicaid cutbacks in the form of reduced eligibility, limits on covered days, and changes in hospital payment combined with implementation of the new Medicare PPS have limited hospital payments from public programs and could therefore alter the distribution of care to the poor.

An Analysis of Hospital Care to the Poor and the Uninsured

The uninsured often face financial barriers when seeking care, and many appear to do without care in the face of such obstacles (Davis and Rowland 1983). For the uninsured who obtain hospital care, access to care can often be limited to a few providers. In part this reflects where the uninsured and the poor live and seek medical care, but it also reflects differences in hospital policies regarding treatment of the uninsured. Some hospitals discourage the uninsured from seeking care by requiring substantial upfront deposits as a condition for admission and limiting access to outpatient services.

The hospital's mix of public and private patients is an important measure of the hospital's ability to subsidize the care of the uninsured from other sources. The proportion of hospital care provided to the uninsured on an inpatient basis provides a rough measure of the hospital's uncompensated care burden, because those who are without insurance coverage are likely to be unable to pay their full hospital bills. However, the scope of uncompensated care is overstated by use of the percentage of admissions without insurance, since some portion of the cost of care for the uninsured is in fact paid directly by the uninsured individuals or their families as a result of hospital collection efforts. Although two-thirds of the uninsured are poor or near-poor, the remaining one-third may be able to pay some portion of their bill.

In this section, patterns of inpatient hospital care for the uninsured and Medicaid population are examined using data from the 1981 Short-Term General and Other Special Hospital Civil Rights Survey, conducted by the Office of Civil Rights of the Department of Health and Human Services, and from the 1980–84 AHA annual surveys. The Civil Rights Survey provides information on inpatient admissions by source of payment for all hospitals treating Medicare or Medicaid patients. It is the only data base available that permits analysis of hospital admissions for the uninsured by proprietary hospitals.

Distribution of Care to the Poor and the Uninsured

The uninsured accounted for 7 percent of all admissions to U.S. hospitals in 1981 (see table 9.1). Medicaid was the primary source of payment for 10 percent of all admissions. Together, uninsured admissions and admissions for the poor with Medicaid accounted for 17 percent of all hospital inpatient admissions. Medicare was the primary source of payment for almost all individuals over age sixty-five and accounted for 33 percent of all admissions. Private insurance and other financing sources accounted for nearly half (49 percent) of hospital admissions.

When the distribution of patient days by source of payment is examined with regard to hospital control, public hospitals had a greater share of their total admissions for uninsured and Medicaid patients than did private hospitals. In large public hospitals with three hundred or more beds, over 19 percent of total admissions were for uninsured patients, compared with 10 percent in small public hospitals, 6 percent in nonprofit hospitals, and 5 percent in for-profit hospitals. Large public hospitals provided three times as much of their care to the uninsured as private hospitals.

The proportion of total patients with Medicaid coverage was more consistent across hospitals but was greatest for large public hospitals. Medicaid patients represented 15 percent of all large public hospital ad-

Table 9.1. **Percentage Distribution of Inpatient Admissions by Source of Payment for Selected Hospital Characteristics, 1981**

Hospital Characteristic	Number of Hospitals	Percentage Total	Uninsured	Medicaid	Medicare	Private/ Others
Ownership						
Nonprofit	3,000	100.0	6.2	9.5	32.2	52.1
For-profit	639	100.0	5.1	10.7	33.4	50.8
Public, small	1,540	100.0	9.6	9.6	36.0	44.7
Public, large	135	100.0	18.7	14.7	22.5	44.2
Bed size						
Fewer than 100	2,481	100.0	8.0	9.8	37.1	45.1
100–299	1,929	100.0	6.5	9.9	30.8	52.9
300–499	626	100.0	7.0	9.2	28.1	55.6
500 or more	278	100.0	9.0	10.7	26.4	53.9
Teaching status						
Nonteaching	4,552	100.0	7.3	9.3	34.1	49.3
Minor teaching	655	100.0	6.8	11.6	28.4	53.2
Major teaching	107	100.0	13.8	20.4	22.0	43.9
Residence						
SMSA	2,640	100.0	6.4	10.6	29.9	53.1
Non-SMSA	2,674	100.0	8.3	9.1	36.4	46.2
Region						
South	1,945	100.0	8.6	9.2	35.0	47.2
West	959	100.0	9.3	12.3	29.7	48.7
Northeast	814	100.0	5.1	10.5	31.9	52.6
North-central	1,596	100.0	5.9	8.7	33.8	51.7
Medicaid generosity by income standard						
Less than 40% of poverty	1,423	100.0	8.7	9.0	35.7	46.6
40–60% of poverty	1,969	100.0	6.9	8.9	31.9	52.3
Above 60% of poverty	1,873	100.0	6.5	11.7	32.7	49.1
Total, all hospitals	5,314	100.0	7.4	9.8	33.2	49.6

Source: Rowland 1987.

missions. Medicaid admissions accounted for 10 percent of total admissions in small public and nonprofit hospitals and 11 percent of admissions in for-profit hospitals.

Thus, the hospitals bearing the greatest burden of care to both the poor on Medicaid and the uninsured were the large public hospitals with over three hundred beds. Over one-third of all admissions to these hospitals were for poor or uninsured patients. Because the proportion of care to the poor and the uninsured is so substantial, these hospitals have the least ability to recover uncovered costs from other third-party payers.

Having a major teaching program for the training of interns and residents was characteristic of hospitals providing a high volume of care to the poor and the uninsured. The 107 hospitals in this analysis with major medical resident training programs (defined as comprising more than 0.25 residents per hospital bed) had the highest proportion of total admissions for uninsured and Medicaid patients. The uninsured constituted 14 percent of all inpatient admissions to major teaching hospitals—a rate almost twice that of minor teaching and nonteaching hospitals. Hospitals with minor teaching programs (defined as comprising fewer than 0.25 residents per hospital bed) did not differ significantly from hospitals without teaching programs in their proportion of care to the uninsured.

Major teaching hospitals also provided a greater share of their care to poor Medicaid patients. Medicaid admissions accounted for 20 percent of all major teaching hospital admissions, in contrast to 12 percent for minor teaching hospitals and 9 percent for nonteaching hospitals. The combination of Medicaid and uninsured admissions accounted for 34 percent of all major teaching hospital admissions.

Hospitals in metropolitan areas had a lower proportion of total admissions that were uninsured and a higher proportion that were Medicaid patients than hospitals in nonmetropolitan areas. Nonmetropolitan areas had a higher proportion of total admissions for Medicare patients (36 percent) than did urban areas (30 percent), reflecting the higher proportion of the elderly population living in rural areas.

Uninsured patients represent a slightly higher proportion of total patients in hospitals in the West and South than in the Northeast and North Central areas. This distribution reflects the distribution of the uninsured population and the greater lack of insurance in the South and West, due both to higher poverty levels and more small employers, who are less likely to offer private insurance to their employees. Medicaid admissions accounted for 12 percent of total admissions in the West and 11 percent of admissions in the Northeastern. Medicaid patients represented 9 percent of admissions both in the South and in the North Central region. These regional differences reflect differences in poverty rates by region, as well as variations in the scope of Medicaid coverage among states.

The Medicaid eligibility income standard is a major factor governing the percentage of the poor covered by Medicaid. In states where the Medicaid income eligibility level is high and set close to the poverty level, many of the poor are likely to be covered by Medicaid. At the time of the Civil Rights Survey in January 1981 the federal poverty level was $8,414 for a family of four. Ten states set their income eligibility level for Medicaid at less than 40 percent of the poverty level; twenty-one states set theirs at 40–60 percent of the poverty level; and nineteen states set theirs at above 60 percent.

Nationwide, the proportion of care to the poor and the uninsured represents about 18 percent of all inpatient admissions. However, the distribution of care between the poor with Medicaid and the uninsured varies according to the generosity of Medicaid coverage in the state where the hospital is located. Hospitals located in states with income levels for Medicaid below 40 percent of poverty had 9 percent of their admissions for Medicaid patients and 9 percent for uninsured patients. In contrast, hospitals located in states with income levels for Medicaid in excess of 60 percent of poverty had 12 percent of admissions for Medicaid patients and only 7 percent for uninsured patients.

High-Volume Providers of Care to the Uninsured

The proportion of total hospital admissions for uninsured patients varies not only among types of hospitals but also by individual hospitals within each group. Within each group a few hospitals bear a disproportionate share of the care of the uninsured. As shown in table 9.2, 3 percent of all hospitals had high levels (defined as more than 25 percent of all admissions) of uninsured patients. In these 168 hospitals, more than one out of every four patients was without insurance. In contrast, in nearly half of all hospitals fewer than 5 percent of total admissions were uninsured. The ability to recover costs for the uninsured through cost shifting to other payers is obviously an easier task for the hospitals in the latter group than in the former. These low-volume uninsured care hospitals are also more likely to be price-competitive because they have less indigent care to cross-subsidize.

Although public hospitals generally have higher indigent care loads than other hospitals, some public hospitals have a much more substantial commitment than others. Seven percent of all public hospitals had over 25 percent of all admissions for uninsured patients. On the other hand, 31 percent of public hospitals had fewer than 5 percent of total admissions for the uninsured, demonstrating the variation in care to the uninsured at the individual hospital level and the uneven burdens for care of uninsured patients even among public hospitals.

The most striking burden for care of the uninsured fell on the large public hospitals with three hundred or more beds. Of the 135 hospitals in this category, one-quarter had more than 25 percent of their total admissions for uninsured patients. Even small public hospitals, with less than three hundred beds, were more likely to be high-volume providers to the uninsured than were for-profit or nonprofit hospitals. In 1981, 6 percent of small public hospitals had uninsured admissions in excess of 25 percent of total admissions, in contrast to less than 2 percent of either nonprofit or for-profit hospitals.

Among the hospitals with major teaching programs, 18 percent had

Table 9.2. **Percentage of Hospitals with More Than 25 Percent or Fewer Than 5 Percent of Total Admissions for the Uninsured, by Selected Characteristics, 1981**

Hospital Characteristic	Number of Hospitals	Uninsured Admissions as Percentage of All Admissions	
		Fewer than 5%	More than 25%
Ownership			
Nonprofit	3,000	51.7	1.2
For-profit	639	64.9	1.7
Public	1,675	31.3	7.2
Public, small	1,540	32.7	5.6
Public, large	135	15.6	25.2
Bed size			
Fewer than 100	2,481	42.1	3.5
100–299	1,929	51.9	2.2
300–499	626	52.2	3.7
500 or more	278	41.7	5.8
Teaching status			
Nonteaching	4,552	45.6	2.7
Minor teaching	655	56.9	3.8
Major teaching	107	36.4	17.8
Residence			
SMSA	2,640	57.5	3.1
Non-SMSA	2,674	36.3	3.3
Medicaid Income Standards, 1980			
Less than 40% of poverty	1,423	38.9	4.6
40–60% of poverty	1,969	48.8	2.7
Above 60% of poverty	1,873	51.4	2.2
Total	5,314	46.8	3.2

Source: Rowland 1987.

more than 25 percent of their patients uninsured, but in 36 percent fewer than 5 percent were without insurance. Only 3 percent of nonteaching hospitals and 4 percent of minor teaching hospitals had a high proportion of uninsured patients.

A high volume of care to the uninsured was more likely to be a problem for hospitals in states with restrictive Medicaid eligibility levels. Of the hospitals located in states with Medicaid income levels below 40 percent of the federal poverty level, 5 percent had more than 25 percent of their admissions for uninsured patients. In the more liberal eligibility states, with income standards over 60 percent of the poverty level, only 2 percent of hospitals had over 25 percent of total admissions for the uninsured.

Table 9.3. Comparison of All Hospitals with Hospitals Having More Than 25 Percent of Total Admissions for the Uninsured, by Selected Characteristics, 1981

Hospital Characteristic	All Hospitals (N = 5,314)	High-Volume Hospitals (N = 168)
	Percentage Distribution	
Ownership	100.00	100.00
Nonprofit	56.50	22.00
For-profit	12.00	6.60
Public, small	29.00	51.20
Public, large	2.50	20.20
Bed Size	100.00	100.00
Fewer than 100	46.70	51.80
100–299	36.30	25.00
300–499	11.80	13.70
500 or more	5.20	9.50
Teaching status	100.00	100.00
Nonteaching	85.70	73.80
Minor teaching	12.30	14.90
Major teaching	2.00	11.30
Residence	100.00	100.00
SMSA	49.70	48.20
Non-SMSA	50.30	51.80
Medicaid Income Standards, 1980	100.00	100.00
Less than 40% of poverty	27.00	40.40
40–60% of poverty	37.40	33.50
More than 60% of poverty	35.60	26.10

Source: Rowland 1987.

As shown in table 9.3, public hospitals are more likely than either nonprofit or for-profit hospitals to be high-volume providers to the uninsured. Public hospitals represent 31 percent of all hospitals but 71 percent of high-volume providers to the uninsured. Major teaching hospitals represent 2 percent of all hospitals but account for 11 percent of high-volume hospitals by teaching status. Finally, hospitals in states with low Medicaid income standards (standards below 40 percent of the poverty level) constitute 27 percent of all hospitals but 40 percent of high-volume providers to the uninsured.

The burden of care for the uninsured is thus a significant problem for a small group of hospitals. Of the 5,314 hospitals analyzed here, 37 nonprofit, 11 for-profit, and 120 public hospitals had over 25 percent of their admissions for the uninsured. The 168 facilities in this situation are most likely to be the hospitals under financial stress from efforts to contain costs by limiting payments to hospitals under Medicare, Medicaid, and employer health plans.

Summary

In summary, when the distribution of care to the uninsured and Medicaid population is examined by hospital characteristics, ownership and teaching status are identified as the most significant indicators of a hospital's likelihood of caring for a high proportion of uninsured and Medicaid patients. Public hospitals and teaching hospitals have a greater share of their total care for Medicaid and uninsured patients than do private hospitals and nonteaching hospitals. Non-profit hospitals provide a higher proportion of total care to the uninsured than do for-profit hospitals, but for Medicaid their proportion of total care is similar.

However, the region in which the hospital is located and the scope of Medicaid coverage of the poor in the state also appear to be important factors. Hospitals in the more generous Medicaid states have a lower proportion of total care for the uninsured than do hospitals located in states where Medicaid coverage is more restrictive. Bed size and location in an SMSA do not appear to be strong determinants of the distribution of care.

Changes in Medicaid Inpatient Hospital Admissions, 1980–1984

Medicaid cost containment policies were implemented in most states during the 1980–85 period as a result of cutbacks in federal funding enacted in the Omnibus Budget Reconciliation Act of 1981. As described in chapter 4, eligibility for Medicaid among families with dependent children was reduced, and many states developed their own payment methods for hospital care and began to exercise new flexibility with regard to program design and beneficiaries' freedom to choose their provider. These policy changes have affected both hospitals' willingness to care for Medicaid patients and the size of the uninsured poor population seeking care. This section looks at Medicaid admissions as a proportion of total admissions in 1980 as compared with 1984 in order to assess the impact of state Medicaid cost containment policies on hospital utilization by the Medicaid-covered poor.

In 1980 Medicaid admissions accounted for 11 percent of all hospital admissions. By 1984 the share of total admissions for Medicaid patients had dropped to 10 percent. As shown in table 9.4, Medicaid admissions decreased by 7 percent over the five-year-period, while total hospital admissions decreased by only 3 percent. The decline in Medicaid admissions accounted for 25 percent of the decline in total admissions.

The most notable change in Medicaid admissions from 1980 to 1984

Table 9.4. Percentage of Medicaid Admissions and Percentage Change in Medicaid and Total Admissions for Selected Hospital Characteristics, 1980 and 1984

Hospital Characteristic	Number of Hospitals	Percentage Medicaid Admissions		Percentage Change in Medicaid Admissions	Percentage Change in Total Admissions
		1980	1984		
Control					
Nonprofit	2,773	9.9	9.4	−7.4	−2.8
For-profit	542	8.3	6.1	−30.4	−4.4
Public	1,450	13.5	13.8	−1.2	−3.0
Public, small	1,324	10.7	10.9	−3.5	−5.5
Public, large	126	18.3	18.2	1.1	1.2
Bed size					
Fewer than 100	2,090	10.4	9.9	−11.9	−8.1
100–299	1,774	10.0	9.4	−8.8	−3.1
300–499	610	9.9	9.4	−8.0	−2.5
500 or more	291	12.0	11.7	−2.2	−0.4
Teaching status					
Nonteaching	3,673	8.9	8.5	−8.2	−4.3
Minor teaching	987	10.6	10.0	−8.7	−2.5
Major teaching	105	22.0	20.8	−0.7	4.8
Residence					
SMSA	2,433	10.8	10.1	−8.4	−2.0
Non-SMSA	2,332	9.5	9.8	−3.2	−6.2
Region					
Northeast	813	12.5	12.2	−1.0	1.2
North-central	1,462	9.9	10.2	−5.1	−8.1
South	1,649	8.4	7.8	−9.4	−2.1
West	841	12.7	10.7	−17.3	−1.6
Total	4,765	10.5	10.0	−7.3	−3.0

Source: Rowland 1987.

was the drop in Medicaid admissions in for-profit hospitals. During this period the total volume of admissions in for-profit hospitals decreased by 4 percent, but Medicaid admissions fell 30 percent. Medicaid patients accounted for over half of the total decline in admissions in for-profit hospitals. In 1980, 8 percent of all admissions to for-profit hospitals were for Medicaid patients; by 1984 the figure was only 6 percent.

The decline in Medicaid admissions in nonprofit hospitals also outstripped the decline in total admissions, but the effect was not as dramatic as the change in for-profit facilities. Medicaid admissions in nonprofit hospitals decreased by 7 percent from 1980 to 1984, while total admissions decreased by 3 percent. As a result, nonprofit hospitals' share of total admissions for Medicaid patients dropped from 10 percent in 1980 to 9 percent in 1984.

Public hospitals, on the other hand, slightly increased their share of total admissions for Medicaid patients during the period from 13.5 percent in 1980 to 13.8 percent in 1984. Total Medicaid admissions in public hospitals declined by 1 percent over this period, but the share of admissions for Medicaid increased, because the decline in Medicaid admissions was more moderate than the 3 percent decline in total admissions.

The only ownership group for which Medicaid admissions increased over this time was large public hospitals with over three hundred beds. Medicaid admissions in these hospitals increased by 1 percent, but the total volume of care to all patients also increased slightly during this period. As a result, the share of total admissions for Medicaid patients remained relatively stable at 18 percent.

The total volume of care in hospitals with large teaching programs increased by 5 percent from 1980 to 1984, but the number of Medicaid admissions decreased slightly. As a result, Medicaid admissions as a proportion of total admissions decreased from 22 percent in 1980 to 21 percent in 1984. Medicaid admissions in minor teaching hospitals and nonteaching hospitals also fell more rapidly than overall admissions during this period. Medicaid admissions declined by 9 percent in minor teaching hospitals and 8 percent in nonteaching hospitals, while overall admissions in these facilities declined by 3 percent and 4 percent, respectively.

The decline in Medicaid admissions was greater in hospitals in SMSAs than in hospitals in non-SMSAs. In SMSAs, Medicaid admissions decreased by 8 percent, while overall admissions decreased by 2 percent. In non-SMSAs the decline in Medicaid admissions was 3 percent, while overall admissions decreased by 6 percent. Because Medicaid admissions declined less than overall admissions in non-SMSAs, the proportion of total admissions for Medicaid patients in hospitals in non-SMSAs increased slightly, from 9.5 percent in 1980 to 9.8 percent in 1984. These findings suggest that Medicaid patients are becoming a more important component of the patient base for hospitals in non-SMSAs as the overall volume of patients declines. Traditionally, Medicaid coverage has been most extensive in urban areas, because eligibility is keyed to single-parent families, which are more prevalent in urban areas. This analysis points to the growing importance of Medicaid as a source of patients and revenue for hospitals outside the SMSAs.

By region, the most notable change in Medicaid admissions occurred in the West, where Medicaid admissions declined by 17 percent. In contrast to the drop in Medicaid admissions, total admissions in the West declined by only 2 percent. Medicaid admissions as a proportion of total admissions dropped from 13 percent in 1980 to 11 percent in 1984. There was also a notable decline in Medicaid admissions in the South, where Medicaid admissions dropped by 9 percent, compared with a 2 percent drop in overall admissions. These regional trends reflect differences in Medicaid policies in the various states comprising each region, as well as other factors related to the economy and functioning of the hospital industry in the state where the hospital is located.

In sum, among hospitals, the for-profit hospitals appear to have had the most radical reduction in care to Medicaid patients. This may reflect the ability of the for-profit hospitals to respond quickly to changing policies because of their corporate structure. If for-profit hospitals are reducing their care to the Medicaid population, they will be more insulated from Medicaid policy changes and can rely more on private patients as a revenue base.

This shift in care burdens has implications for access to care for the Medicaid population and could significantly affect the future fiscal viability of public hospitals. If the concentration of admissions for Medicaid patients increases in the public hospitals and decreases in private hospitals, the Medicaid goal of mainstream medical care for the poor could be lost. Instead, Medicaid patients increasingly would be cared for in public hospitals.

If public hospitals have a higher proportion of patients on Medicaid because patients that previously would have been treated in the for-profit or non-profit hospitals are now shifted to public hospitals for their care, public hospitals will be more directly influenced by Medicaid policies. Cost containment policies under Medicaid will have a more serious impact on the public hospitals than on private hospitals.

Protecting the Poor and Sick in a Cost-conscious Society

The need to improve health care coverage for the uninsured has resurfaced as a priority as the number of uninsured Americans continues to climb and cost containment pressures adversely affect the providers of care to the poor and uninsured. Budget cuts at the federal and state levels are constraining Medicaid hospital payments and leading hospitals to be wary of providing a high volume of care to the poor (AHA 1982). Limits on Medicaid have made the indigent care problems worse in many states.

Thirty-seven million Americans, or 17 percent of the non-aged population, were not covered by public or private insurance plans in 1986 (Census 1987a). The lack of insurance is a difficult problem particularly for low-income Americans because they have the least ability to pay for unexpected health care problems. Although Medicaid finances medical care for many low-income Americans, and some individuals are privately insured through their employers, over one-third of the poor—12.6 million people—were uninsured in 1984 (Sulvetta and Swartz 1986).

The growing concern for the uninsured is intertwined with increasing concern for the financial viability of the institutions that serve the poor. Hospitals with a heavy care burden for indigent patients are more likely to be financially stressed than institutions with a lower indigent care proportion (Mulstein 1984). As cost containment pressure mounts and the uninsured population grows, many of these institutions may be forced to restrict care to the poor in order to survive.

Even in an era of cost containment, the problem of the uninsured, especially the poor and uninsured, cannot be ignored. Efforts to contain health care spending will only intensify their plight and increase the burden on the few hospitals that provide a substantial amount of care to this vulnerable population. A comprehensive cost containment approach should also address the financing of care for the uninsured.

Chapter 10   **The Impact of Cost Containment Efforts on the Quality of Care**

$\mathbf{O}$ver the past decade numerous strategies have been pursued in an effort to decrease or at least control the rate of increase in health care spending. Most prominent among these have been the DRG-based PPS implemented by Medicare in 1983 and capitated systems of care, such as HMOs, which have proliferated in recent years. While these payment reforms provide desirable incentives with respect to health care spending, simultaneously they offer incentives that could jeopardize the quality of health care provided in this country. Concerns that cost containment efforts could contribute, or already are contributing, to deteriorations in the quality of U.S. health care are in fact becoming more prominent.

The purpose of this chapter is to consider both the potential and the actual relationship between recent cost containment efforts and quality of care and to identify related issues that are most deserving of attention in the coming years. The chapter begins with a consideration of how quality of care should be construed and measured. An assessment of the theoretical relationship between any type of cost containment effort and quality of care follows. We then consider the potential quality of care impacts of DRG-based prospective hospital payment and capitation, the mechanisms that have been put into place to ensure quality of care under these two innovative systems of payment, and the actual quality of care experience with them to date.

What Is Quality?

To determine the impact of cost containment efforts on the quality of health care, one needs to begin by defining what quality is and how it is to be measured. The standard dimensions along which quality of care is now assessed consist of Donabedian's classic triad: the structure, process, and outcome of health care services (Donabedian 1980). *Structure* refers to inputs into health care, such as the number, size, and character

200

of hospital facilities, the types of technologies available for use in those facilities, and the mix and qualifications of physician and nonphysician providers that are utilized in the process of delivering health care. *Process* refers to the patterns with which these inputs are employed. Thus, hospital admission and readmission rates, length of hospital stay, and the frequency with which various diagnostic and therapeutic services are utilized are all measures of the process of care. *Outcome*, in turn, refers to the net result of use of health care services on the well-being of individuals. Mortality rates, procedure complication rates, and patients' functional and overall health status are examples of the types of outcome measures that could be used to evaluate the quality of care.

Although structure, process, and outcome measures can provide an indication of the quality of care, they are neither precise nor complete descriptors of quality. An increase or decrease in the number of hospital beds, for example, does not necessarily reflect an improvement or deterioration in quality or accessibility of care. Similarly, the relationship between patterns of practice (a process measure) and quality of care is not always clear. In a recent study conducted for the Congressional Office of Technology Assessment, for example, Chassin (1983) found no relationship between variations in hospital length of stay for each of five different medical disorders and the outcomes of those hospitalizations. Wennberg and others (Brook et al. 1984; Chassin et al. 1986; Eddy 1984; Wennberg 1984; Wennberg and Gittlesohn 1975, 1982) have called attention to these variations in practice. In many of these instances there is disagreement within the medical profession itself about the optimal strategy for management of individual medical problems. Thus, it is not clear whether variations in practice reflect underprovision or overprovision of services, or both (Chassin et al. 1986, 1987; Wennberg 1986, 1987). This uncertainty regarding optimal patterns of care is in part due to the fact that our current measures of outcome tend to be crude. In addition, however, medical practice evaluation is complicated by the fact that outcomes are influenced by factors such as individuals' lifestyles, which transcend the health care services that are provided.

Thus, despite the importance of quality of care, our ability to assess quality is poorly developed. As a result, our ability to determine the impact of cost containment efforts on quality of care is also limited. The remainder of this chapter considers what is known about this issue. We begin by considering the potential impacts of cost containment incentives on quality of care. We then review the available data bearing on this issue, the mechanisms that have been put into place to preserve or enhance quality in our era of cost containment, and future directions in policy and research relating to quality.

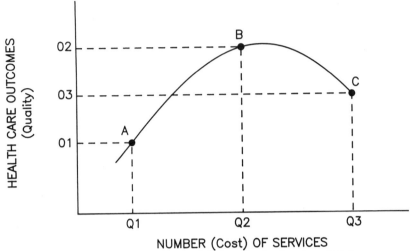

Fig. 10.1 **The Relationship between Health Care Service Inputs and Outcomes**
(*Source:* Chamber of Commerce 1985, p. 31.)

The Potential Impact of Cost Containment on Quality of Care: General Principles

As detailed elsewhere in this book, spending on health care services in this country has increased dramatically over the past two decades. Although this increase in spending has clearly been associated with provision of a more technologically sophisticated style of care, many health care analysts have questioned whether health care outcomes have actually been improved by the spending increases, or whether any improvements that have occurred have been worth the spending increases that have generated them. The cost-based system of reimbursement under which we operated prior to 1983 is considered to have been inflationary and to have given providers little incentive to utilize health care services in an efficient or cost-effective manner. Indeed, in some instances physicians' test-ordering and use of sophisticated, invasive procedures has been thought to have been not only excessive but at times detrimental.

Figure 10.1 depicts a theoretical relationship between the number (or cost) of health services employed and the health care outcomes or quality of care resulting from use of those services. Between Q1 and Q2 increases in service inputs result in improvements in quality of care. The shape of this curve suggests, however, that as one increases service inputs between Q1 and Q2, the marginal benefit derived from the additional resources being deployed decreases. As one increases service inputs even further, to Q3, quality of care actually deteriorates. This decline might result, for example, from unnecessary performance of surgical procedures or from performance of surgery for marginal indications in which the adverse effects of surgery outweigh the attendant benefits. Within this theoretical construct, one could both improve quality and decrease the cost of health care by reducing utilization from Q3 to Q2.

Obviously, the relationship between health care service inputs (or spending) and outcomes is much more complicated than depicted in figure 10.1. The figure suggests, for example, that between Q2 and Q3 every additional service employed produces a decrease in quality of care. It is more likely, however, that at all points between Q1 and Q3 some service inputs result in benefits, others generate costs with few if any improvements in health outcomes, and still others actually contribute to a decline in patient well-being. In *aggregate,* however, an increase in service inputs between Q1 and Q2 results in an improvement in quality, while an increase between Q2 and Q3 results in a deterioration of quality.

Given this theoretical construct, the impact on health care quality of decreases in health care spending can be seen to depend not only on where one is operating at baseline on the curve in figure 10.1 but also, and what is more important, on the particular services that are withdrawn as part of the decreases in spending. If, for example, incentives and the requisite scientific knowledge could be provided to health care providers to enable them to eliminate detrimental services selectively, then health care outcomes could be improved at the same time that spending was being decreased.

In the real world, incentives are not "pure" and scientific knowledge is not perfect. Physicians and other providers try to do what they think is best, without always knowing whether the benefits of their actions outweigh the associated risks and costs. Consequently, in a health care system in which physicians and hospitals are paid more for doing more, and thus in which there is little incentive to restrain spending, physicians and hospitals will provide more services—of which some will be beneficial and some will be of little or no benefit. In a system in which resources for health care services are constrained, in contrast, physicians and hospitals will perforce provide fewer services. Some of the service reductions will have little adverse effect on quality or may even enhance quality. Other service reductions, however, will result in a deterioration of the quality of care, however quality is defined.

It is the fact that increases in health care spending beget waste as well as benefit that has led to public (or at least governmental) pressure to contain health care costs. It is the reciprocal fact that cutbacks in health care spending will in some instances lead to erosions of quality at the same time that waste is eliminated that has generated current concerns about the impact of health care cost containment on the quality of care. It is within the context of this intrinsic tension between incentives for cost control and concerns about erosion of quality that the Medicare DRG-based PPS and capitated systems of care, such as HMOs, are considered in the next two sections.

DRG-based Prospective Payment

Theory

The DRG-based PPS implemented for Medicare in 1983 was designed to provide physicians and hospitals with incentives to improve the efficiency and cost-effectiveness of health care services provided to hospitalized Medicare beneficiaries. Because savings derived from caring for patients at a cost that is less than the DRG payment rate devolves to hospitals as "profit," and because cost overruns derived from caring for patients at a cost that is greater than the DRG payment rate devolves to hospitals as a "loss," the same incentive that operates to induce hospitals to provide care efficiently may also induce them to skimp on the services they provide. It is difficult at this point to determine what balance will be struck between these two potential outcomes.

Table 10.1 lists a number of *potential* impacts of the DRG-based PPS on structure, access, process, and outcomes of care. There is every reason to expect that PPS will induce a number of beneficial changes in our health care system. Hospital management information systems, utilization review programs, and quality assurance programs will likely be improved. Excess hospital beds will be eliminated, and hospital personnel staffing patterns will be better matched to their needs. Manufacturers, in turn, will place increased emphasis on the development of technologies and therapies that enable physicians to provide care in a more cost-efficient manner. In addition, physician and nonphysician researchers will place increased emphasis on the identification of more cost-effective patterns of practice.

Not all changes induced by PPS will enhance the quality or cost-effectiveness of care, however. For example, under PPS, hospitals have little incentive to acquire new technologies that improve the quality of care, albeit at increased cost (Anderson and Steinberg 1984b; Davis, Anderson, and Steinberg 1984). Were an artificial hip to become available that was more costly but longer-lasting than existing alternatives, for example, hospitals would have little incentive to utilize this technological improvement under PPS (Anderson and Steinberg 1984b). Moreover, given the incentive under PPS to discharge patients as early as possible, some patients will likely be discharged prematurely, leading to either poor outcomes or increased hospital readmission rates (Anderson and Steinberg 1984a).

As predicted by our earlier theoretical discussion, one can expect both beneficial and adverse results to occur. In some instances, moreover, whether the net effect of changes in practice induced by PPS is beneficial or injurious to patients will depend on the accessibility of out-of-hospital services that are substituted for in-hospital care and the availability of third-party insurance to cover their use. Consider, for example, a patient with endocarditis (an infection of a heart valve). Traditionally, physicians have treated endocarditis with four to six weeks of in-hospital intravenous antibiotics. During the last four to five weeks of this treatment many patients are quite stable and have in the past been hospitalized primarily in order to receive antibiotics intravenously rather than because of a need for constant physician oversight.

Given advances in the equipment used to administer medications intravenously, many patients can now complete their course of intravenous antibiotic treatment at home. Moreover, in some instances stable patients who adequately absorb oral antibiotics can be treated at home with oral rather than intravenous therapy. By means of either of these options the cost of treatment can be reduced markedly. PPS provides an incentive to use these alternative treatments. For many patients, home treatment is preferable to hospital confinement as long as home treatment and occasional outpatient follow-up visits are covered by Medicare. Thus, were Medicare to cover these equipment, medication, and physician outpatient visit costs, and were only those patients selected for home treatment who were knowledgeable and motivated enough to employ it, high-quality care could be maintained at decreased cost. On the other hand, were patients forced to pay for these services on their own (current Medicare practice), and were patients who were unable to administer their own therapy or who were not motivated enough to comply with their therapeutic regimen placed on home therapy as part of a new treatment routine, quality of care and patient satisfaction would decrease. Thus, while PPS has the ability to induce changes in practice that maintain or enhance quality of care, it also provides incentives that could result in erosions of the quality of care through efforts to contain costs.

Data

Since PPS has only been in effect since 1983, minimal data exist upon which to base conclusions about its impact on quality of care. In addition, it is unlikely that changes in health care practices that have occurred since 1983 can be attributed solely to implementation of PPS (Davis et al. 1985). Nonetheless it is worth reviewing what little data exist.

Contrary to what one would have predicted given the incentives im-

Table 10.1. **Potential Impacts of DRG-based Prospective Payment on the Quality of Health Care**

Type of Changes	Potential Impact		
	Positive	*Negative*	*Positive and Negative*
Structural changes	Reduced excess hospital bed capacity	Decreased investment in technologies that improve patient care but increase its cost	Increased specialization of service provision
	Improved hospital management information systems and strategies	Failure of some hospitals for reasons other than low efficiency (e.g., attraction of disproportionate share of patients who are severely ill or lack ability to pay)	Diversification of services offered by hospitals
	Improved hospital utilization review and quality assurance programs		Increase in type and volume of outpatient services
Changes in access	Increased availability of services outside of hospitals	Decreased ability to use outpatient services intended to substitute for inpatient services, due to either lack of availability of those services or increased patient cost-sharing in the outpatient sector	Increased service specialization may improve quality of services being offered but reduce availability of full range of services
		Reduced willingness of hospitals to provide charity care	
		Decreased availability of some cost-increasing technologies and services	

Changes in process	Decreased use of unnecessary diagnostic and therapeutic services Improvements in coordination of health care services	Premature hospital discharge in effort to reduce costs Inappropriate triage of high-risk patients to outpatient surgery and procedure centers Decreased length of stay prior to elective surgery leading, in some instances, to poor outcomes and less patient teaching, understanding, and satisfaction	Earlier transfer from acute-care hospitals to rehabilitation hospitals, nursing homes, and home care
Changes in outcome	Reduced risk of nosocomial infections and procedural complications due to shorter lengths of hospital stays and decreased use of unnecessary diagnostic and therapeutic procedures	Increases in morbidity and mortality due to decreased use of beneficial but cost-increasing diagnostic and therapeutic procedures Increases in morbidity, mortality, and patient/family stress due to inadequacy of home care services following earlier hospital discharge.	

Sources: Derived in part from Lewin and Associates 1986; and Lohr et al. 1985.

plicit in PPS, the number of admissions of individuals sixty-five years of age or older to nonfederal acute-care hospitals decreased from 11.8 million in 1983 to 10.8 million in 1987, a decrease of 8.5 percent (HCFA 1988). HCFA has reported a lower rate of decline in admissions among the very elderly (age eighty-five or older) than among those aged sixty-five to sixty-nine (Eggers 1985). This decline in admission rates has not been limited to Medicare beneficiaries, however. Hospital admissions for patients under sixty-five years of age decreased from 25.9 million in 1983 to 22.8 million in 1987, a decrease of 12 percent. Lengths of hospital stay have also declined for patients sixty-five years of age or older, from 9.7 days in 1983 to 8.9 days in 1987. For patients under age sixty-five, the average length of hospital stay dropped from 5.8 days in 1983 to 5.6 days in 1987 (HCFA 1988).

The combination of decreases in admission rates and lengths of stay resulted in a decline in community hospital occupancy rates from 74 percent in 1983 to 64 percent in 1986 (AHA 1987). As one would expect, these decreases in hospital admission rates and lengths of stay have been accompanied by sharp increases in the number of outpatient visits. Outpatient visits to hospitals, for example, increased from 229 million in 1983 to 279 million in 1987 (HCFA 1988). Early data indicate that the increase predicted in hospital readmission rates under PPS (Anderson and Steinberg 1984a) has not occurred (Eggers 1985). Nor is there any indication that either in-hospital or out-of-hospital mortality rates have increased under PPS.

This "standard fare" of process data provides little indication of the actual impact of PPS on either patient outcomes or overall quality of care, however. Sixty-six percent of 389 physicians responding to a survey conducted by the AMA, however, believe that the quality of patient care has deteriorated under PPS as a result of increased pressure to discharge patients earlier and earlier (AMA 1985). The American Society of Internal Medicine has also reported an indication from physicians that pressure from hospital administrators has led to premature discharges and that necessary out-of-hospital care frequently is not available to patients after their hospitalization (American Society of Internal Medicine 1985).

The U.S. Senate Committee on Aging has also reported disturbing anecdotal indications that in some instances the incentives implicit in PPS have engendered quite undesirable patterns of medical practice. The committee conducted a four-month investigation of the impact of PPS on the quality of care received by Medicare beneficiaries (Senate Special Committee on Aging 1985). Committee staff visited and collected data from five PROs and several community and university hospitals. The inquiry included interviews with Medicare beneficiaries, physicians and nurses, researchers, and personnel from PROs, hospitals, HCFA, and the Department of Health and Human Services Office of the Inspector General. The committee identified four major problem areas:

- Seriously ill Medicare patients are being discharged prematurely from hospitals.
- Hospitalized patients frequently are too sick to appeal hospital discharge decisions and lack adequate protection under Medicare's PPS.
- Many patients, especially the terminally ill, and their families are being given incomplete and at times inaccurate information regarding their coverage benefits and options for posthospital care.
- Some hospitals appear to have denied admission to patients with multiple or serious conditions because of a concern that those patients would generate losses under PPS.

More recently, the DHHS Inspector General conducted a comprehensive review of the care provided to hospitalized Medicare beneficiaries in an effort to identify cases of premature discharge and inappropriate transfers. In this analysis the Inspector General reviewed 3,549 problem cases reported to HCFA by PROs. The study identified 2,149 cases of poor quality care, ranging from minor deficiencies to patients who did not receive necessary routine tests or who were prematurely discharged or had to be readmitted because of their inability to manage at home following discharge (Kusserow 1986).

Although there is no indication that these types of abuses are occurring on a widespread basis (researchers at CPHA, for example, found no evidence of deterioration of the quality of care in 729 hospitals during the first year of PPS [DesHarnais et al. 1987]), these anecdotes provide obvious reason for concern and underscore the need for integration of timely and thorough quality assurance mechanisms into PPS. Thus far, however, no scientific study has concluded that quality of care has declined under PPS. Although discharges of patients to skilled-nursing facilities and home health agencies have increased under PPS, whether these discharges have been inappropriate has not been determined (Schramm and Gabel 1988).

Quality Control Mechanisms under PPS

Several mechanisms exist or are being developed in an effort to help assure that the quality of health care is not eroded under PPS. One such mechanism is the Utilization and Quality Control Peer Review Organization (PRO) Program. The PRO program was initiated by Congress in an effort to monitor hospital use and quality of care provided to Medicare patients under PPS. When HCFA issued a request for proposals from PRO applicants in February 1984, it defined a number of cost, utilization, and quality control objectives that it wanted PROs to meet. Cost and utilization objectives included reductions in admissions for procedures that could be performed safely on an outpatient basis, reductions in inappropriate admissions and use of unnecessary ancillary services, and elimination of inappropriate cardiac pacemaker implantations or reimplantations. Quality control objectives included reductions in inappropriate transfers from one PPS hospital to another, unnecessary hospital readmissions resulting from substandard care during the preceding admission, avoidable deaths, unnecessary surgery or other invasive procedures, and avoidable postoperative and other complications (Dans, Weiner, and Otter 1985).

PROs were also asked to ensure that essential medical services (i.e., those without which there is a potential for serious complications) were provided. The fifty-four local PROs approved by HCFA in 1984 were expected to achieve these objectives through retrospective reviews of hospital records and discharge abstract data combined with education of physicians regarding deficiencies, recommendations for denials of payment for inappropriate care, and use of sanctions (e.g., termination from participation in the Medicare program) for hospitals or physicians failing to meet professionally recognized standards of care (Dans, Weiner, and Otter 1985).

Although the PRO program has been operating only since 1984, concerns have already been voiced that its energies have been inappropriately focused on utilization review and cost containment concerns rather than on quality assurance (Dans, Weiner, and Otter 1985; Senate Special Committee on Aging 1985). For example, the Senate Committee on Aging pointed out that PROs are not expected to review outpatient care, readmissions that occur more than seven days after discharge, failures to provide appropriate discharge planning or follow-up, medical complications that result from denials of hospitalization or refusals by nursing homes to accept patients with aboveaverage nursing care needs (Senate Special Committee on Aging 1985).

In response to these concerns, the American Medical Peer Review Association (AMPRA), a national organization representing PROs and other physician-directed medical review groups, recommended a number of changes in the PRO program, including the development and application of uniform quality and discharge planning screens and expansion of PRO activities beyond the inpatient setting (AMPRA 1985). In addition, in January 1986 HCFA revised the proposed scope of work for PROs in their second two-year contract period so as to ensure increased effort to reduce adverse outcomes, such as premature hospital discharges. In order to identify poor quality care, PROs were asked to apply generic quality screens developed by HCFA to several broad areas of concern: the adequacy of discharge planning, nosocomial infections, unscheduled return to surgery within a single admission for the same condition or to correct an operative problem, trauma suffered in the hospital, and deaths. In addition, PROs have been asked to perform intensive reviews of hospitals and DRGs in which patterns of practice depart markedly from national or local norms, to review readmissions that occur within fifteen (rather than the previous seven) days, and to establish community outreach programs (ProPAC 1986).

In an effort to improve the quality of care under PPS as well as to provide congressional review of that care, Senator Heinz of Pennsylvania and Congressman Stark of California introduced the Medicare quality protection bill, which requires (1) that PROs devote "a reasonable proportion" of their funds to quality care review; (2) that PROs investigate all beneficiary complaints relating to quality of care; (3) that hospitals develop uniform needs assessment instruments to help identify out-of-hospital resources that can be utilized following discharge; and (4) formal discharge planning by hospitals (C. Davis 1986). The last two provisions were included in legislation passed by Congress in 1987. As of April 1987, PROs have been required to review services provided to Medicare beneficiaries by HMOs and CMPs (House Committee on Ways and Means 1988).

In addition to legislative quality control efforts, several other forces operate to assure quality of care under PPS. First, unlike hospitals, physicians are still paid by Medicare on an FFS basis. Thus, although hospital revenues are fixed regardless of patients' length of stay, physicians' payments increase as patients stay in the hospital longer. This divergence between the fiscal incentives confronting hospitals and physicians serves to counterbalance pressure on physicians to discharge patients earlier and earlier. Second, both hospitals and physicians face concerns about malpractice suits and have an obvious interest in doing good work in order to preserve or enhance the number of patients for whom they care. Finally, health services researchers increasingly have been attracted to assessments of the quality of care provided to Medicare beneficiaries under PPS. Under a contract from HCFA, for example, the Rand Corporation has undertaken a study (expected to be completed in 1989) designed to compare the quality of care provided to patients before and after implementation of PPS. Disease-specific process measures, such as the appropriateness of diagnostic and therapeutic services provided to patients, and outcome measures, such as mortality rates and health status at the time of discharge, will be evaluated for common and important medical disorders (Brook and Kahn 1985). This type of attention from health services researchers to quality of care not only should help provide us with insights into the impacts of PPS but may also provide incentives to physicians to maintain high-quality standards of practice.

Capitation

Theory

A second major payment reform intended to reduce health care costs is capitation. Capitated systems of health care, such as HMOs, are increasing in numbers as interest in cost containment intensifies (see chapter 7). HMOs, like hospitals operating under PPS, have incentives to discharge patients from hospitals as early as possible and to utilize as few diagnostic tests, treatments, and ancillary services during a hospitalization as is consistent with good-quality care. Capitated systems offer a number of potential quality and cost-related advantages over DRG-based prospective payment, however, which derive from the fact that they generally are paid for caring for a patient for a year rather than for a single hospitalization. Consequently, unlike hospitals under PPS, capitated systems such as HMOs have no incentive to unbundle multiproblem admissions into multiple admissions (Anderson and Steinberg 1984a) or to hospitalize patients for problems that could be cared for adequately in an outpatient setting. In addition, because of the longer time frame of their financial responsibility, HMOs might be more likely than hospitals operating under PPS to utilize therapeutic services that are cost-saving in the long run but not in the short run (Anderson and Steinberg 1984b) and to prevent avoidable hospital readmissions by ensuring that necessary follow-up services are arranged for patients discharged from the hospital. Thus, one might expect vertical integration or diversification of services within HMOs (e.g., with a single HMO operating an outpatient facility, hospital, skilled nursing facility, and home health service) to facilitate early discharge from hospitals and coordinated care for episodes of illness.

As is the case with hospitals under PPS, the concern with capitated systems is that financial considerations will lead HMOs to underprovide necessary services. In the case of HMOs, however, concerns about underprovision of necessary care apply not only to diagnostic, therapeutic, and ancillary services for hospitalized patients but also to the possibility that HMOs might not hospitalize patients who need inpatient attention and might skimp on provision of necessary outpatient visits or services. These types of concerns are particularly strong because HMO physicians' incomes are directly or indirectly affected by costs generated by the care they provide to their patients. Table 10.2 summarizes some of the potential positive and negative impacts of capitated systems on access to and the structure, process, and outcomes of care.

Data

Studies comparing the quality of care provided in HMOs with that provided in the FFS sector suggest that quality of care in HMOs as a whole is at least as good as and possibly better than that provided in the FFS sector (Cunningham and Williamson 1980; Luft 1981). The evidence available comes from a small number of studies of relatively few HMOs. Almost all HMOs studied were mature group practice or staff model HMOs operating in an environment less focused on competition and cost containment than is the case today (Luft 1988). Because of a belief that HMOs perform fewer diagnostic tests, employ less qualified physicians, and do not allow adequate doctor-patient relationships to develop, some physicians believe that HMOs offer care that is inferior to that provided in the FFS sector. A national survey has provided no evidence that HMO physicians are less skilled than their FFS counterparts, however. Moreover, 90 percent of HMO members are satisfied with the quality of the doctors caring for them (Louis Harris and Associates 1984).

Although data comparing the process of care for specific diseases in HMOs with that in FFS settings are limited, three studies provide some insight into the comparative styles of practice under these two different systems of payment. In the first study, the existence of a population-based cancer registry in a community with an HMO enabled researchers to compare the care given for colorectal cancer in an HMO with that given in the FFS sector (Francis, Polissar, and Lorenz 1984). In this study of 189 patients (39 in the HMO and 150 in FFS practices), HMO providers gave a greater volume of care (e.g., number of physician visits and endoscopies) than FFS providers during the interval from first contact with the patient until the disease was diagnosed and treated. As a result, there was a significantly longer pretreatment interval for HMO patients. Once the diagnosis of colorectal cancer was made, however, there were no differences in rates of definitive surgery, chemotherapy or radiation therapy, lengths of hospital stay, or number of follow-up visits. No differences were found in selfreported health status at three and twelve months or in survival after four years. Despite the belief that HMOs might be more inclined to provide preventive health services (including screening) than FFS providers, the percentage of patients who had their disease detected as a result of routine physical examination or screening procedures, rather than as a result of follow-up of symptoms, was the same in the HMO patients (10 percent) and the FFS patients (12 percent).

In a second study, Yelin et al. (1985) found no significant differences in hospital admission rates, lengths of hospital stay, or rates of surgery between rheumatoid arthritis patients cared for by rheumatologists in HMOs and those cared for by rheumatologists in FFS practices. HMO

Table 10.2. Potential Impacts of Capitation on the Quality of Health Care

Type of Changes	Potential Impact		
	Positive	Negative	Positive and Negative
Structural changes	Reduced excess hospital bed capacity due to decreases in hospital admissions		Substitution of nurse practitioners and physician assistants for physicians
	Improved hospital management information systems and strategies		
	Improved hospital utilization review and quality assurance programs		
Changes in access		Decreased access to health care services for high-risk populations due to selective marketing	Increased volume and use of outpatient services
		Decreased access to inpatient care in effort to reduce costs	
		Exclusion of patients unable to pay capitated premium	
Changes in process	Decreased use of unnecessary diagnostic and therapeutic services	Premature hospital discharges in effort to reduce costs	Earlier transfer from acute-care hospitals to rehabilitation hospitals, nursing homes, and home care
	Improved coordination of inpatient and outpatient health care services	Inappropriate triage of high-risk patients to outpatient surgery and procedure centers in effort to reduce costs	Reduced hospitalization

Changes in outcome	Reduced risk of nosocomial infections and procedural complications due to shorter lengths of hospital stays and decreased use of unnecessary diagnostic and therapeutic procedures	Decreased length of stay prior to elective surgery leading, in some instances, to poor outcomes and less patient teaching, understanding and satisfaction
		Delays in use of expensive but beneficial diagnostic or therapeutic services
		Increases in morbidity and mortality due to decreased use of beneficial but cost-increasing diagnostic and therapeutic incentives
		Increases in morbidity, mortality, and patient/family stress due to inadequacy of home care services following earlier hospital discharge

Sources: Derived in part from Lewin and Associates 1986; and Lohr et al. 1985.

rheumatologists saw their patients less frequently than did FFS rheumatologists, but there was no indication that HMO patients were adversely affected as a result.

Finally, Siu et al. (1988) compared hospital admission rates for HMO and FFS patients. They reported that the rate of discretionary surgery was lower in the HMO setting than in the FFS setting, whereas the rate of nondiscretionary surgery was the same in the two settings. Both discretionary and nondiscretionary medical admission rates were lower in the HMO; however, the authors found no observable adverse effects on the health of HMO patients.

Given the fiscal incentives confronting HMOs, one would expect isolated instances of underprovision of care by HMOs even if HMOs as a whole provide high-quality care. Thus, it is no surprise that Medicare beneficiaries in one Florida HMO complained of inadequate care, long delays for appointments, and unsatisfactory emergency treatment ("HMOs Protecting Senior Citizens" 1986). After an extended investigation by the Department of Health and Human Services, the HMO was dropped from the Medicare program (Iglehart 1987). This type of occurrence suggests a need for some sort of oversight mechanism to ensure that HMOs do not underprovide services out of an interest in saving money.

Quality Control Mechanisms

Several types of quality control mechanisms operate to help assure the quality of care provided by HMOs. In the case of federally qualified HMOs, comprehensive benefit packages are a prerequisite for federal qualification. Each federally qualified HMO must also have an ongoing quality assurance program that stresses health outcomes, provides for review by physicians of the process followed in providing health services, and includes written procedures for taking remedial action when inappropriate or substandard services have been provided (Congress 1973). Systematic reviews of patterns of practice within HMOs do not tend to be conducted at either the federal, state, or local level. The Arizona Health Care Cost Containment System, a Medicaid demonstration project that requires that Medicaid beneficiaries receive health care from prepaid health plans such as HMOs or IPAs and has begun annual statewide quality of care reviews, is an exception (Schaller, Bostrom, and Rafferty 1986). Some states, such as Maryland, do require submission and approval of written quality assurance guidelines as a condition for HMO licensure. And in some states the insurance commission assures that each HMO's premiums seem adequate to cover the benefits being offered and requires that HMOs maintain substantial capital reserves to assure fiscal solvency. These types of regulations are not uniform across states, however.

The most powerful quality assurance mechanism affecting HMOs is the marketplace itself. For this type of quality assurance mechanism to operate satisfactorily, however, enrollees must have a sense of what appropriate patterns of practice should be—a condition that is not easily met. Ideally, uniform quality assurance guidelines and processes would be developed and applied to HMOs, with the results provided to consumers in an easily understood but meaningful fashion.

Conclusion

Efforts to contain health care costs have intensified in the past decade. Major payment reforms intended to decrease health care costs, such as DRG-based PPS and capitated systems of health care, have been implemented and are proliferating. Other types of health care cost containment strategies will surely be developed in the coming decade. As this review demonstrates, these cost containment strategies, while laudable, create incentives that jeopardize the quality of health care. Consequently, it is imperative that efforts to preserve or enhance the quality of health care be pursued in tandem with efforts to contain health care costs. These efforts should include increased research on evaluation of the quality of alternative patterns of practice and on better definition and tools for measurement of health care outcomes.

It is not necessarily the case that the quality of health care in this country will deteriorate as health care cost containment efforts are pursued. Rather, quality of care can be improved at the same time that costs are decreased. In order to achieve this desirable result, however, creative incentives need to be devised, and increased financial support needs to be provided for clinical and health services research, in order to help guide physicians in their choices of which health care services to provide to individual patients and which to forgo. It is only through increased clinical and health services research, and implementation of creative policy and management strategies combined with vigilant attention to quality of care that cost containment efforts will succeed in this country.

Chapter 11 · Major Lessons from the Past Experience

Rapid rates of increase in health care costs have characterized the U.S. health care sector for the past thirty-five years. The reason for these increases is clear: the lack of both effective competition in the health care marketplace and effective public policy to constrain cost increases. The consequences are equally clear: difficulty in obtaining care for those without health insurance, major financial burdens on those with inadequate health insurance, high employee health benefit costs that increase the cost of American products and place them at a competitive disadvantage in international markets, and heavy tax burdens resulting from Medicare and Medicaid outlays financing health care for the elderly, the disabled, and many of the nation's poor.

Health policy leaders in the federal government, state governments, and the private sector have brought considerable ingenuity and talent to bear in developing and implementing health care cost containment initiatives over the last fifteen years. The sum of this experience is in many ways greater than the individual parts. The mosaic these initiatives form depicts a fairly clear picture of what works and what does not work to contain health care costs and the impact alternative approaches have on many other important social goals. The following sections attempt to define the salient lessons this rich experience has to offer.

The Political Basis for Change

The United States has a fragmented health financing system and a fragmented provider payment policy. Medicare finances care for the elderly and the disabled and sets its own policies for payment of hospitals, physicians, and other health care providers. Medicaid finances care for large numbers of the nation's poor and medically indigent; states independently design and implement their own provider payment policies. The great majority of workers and their dependents obtain health insurance coverage through their employers; employers and insurance companies design their own cost containment policies. A handful of states have developed hospital rate-setting programs that review hospital budgets or approve prices charged to all patients.

The fragmentation of health financing and provider payment policy in the United States is not an accident or an oversight; it is the result of deliberate political action. It exists because the medical establishment prefers a fragmented system and has brought enormous political pressure to bear in opposition to any unified system—whether it be a national health insurance plan or cost containment measures that apply nationally to all patients (Starr 1982). The most important lesson to be drawn from this long experience is that the primary barrier to effective health care cost containment in the United States is gaining a political consensus for change.

Where policy action has been mounted to curb rising costs, it has followed this general course:

1. Documentation of the extent of the problem and its consequences

2. General public awareness and public support for change

3. A period of experimentation in which health care providers are afforded an opportunity to develop an effective solution to defined problems without policy intervention

4. Failure of voluntary action to solve the problems, adding economic to political pressures for change

5. Development of provider payment reform policy options that show promise of being effective

Change has not occurred in the absence of crisis. State cost containment initiatives were launched during periods of economic recession when expanding Medicaid outlays could not be met in the face of declines in state sales tax revenues, increases in state outlays for unemployment compensation, and other expenditures. The only period of nationwide controls on the health sector occurred during the Nixon Economic Stabilization Program, when inflation in the economy triggered by the Vietnam War was viewed as so serious as to warrant nationwide wage and price controls. Employers began aggressively implementing health care cost containment measures only when faced with extraordinary increases in health insurance premiums at a time of declining sales and intense competition from foreign producers. Reform of Medicare hospital payment also took place in an environment of massive federal budgetary deficits and rapid rates of increase in hospital expenditures and Medicare budgetary outlays.

As a result of these continual responses to crises, the cost containment initiatives have become fragmented, frequently undesirable from a public policy perspective, and often counterproductive when undertaken in combination with other initiatives. For example, Medicaid has suppressed physician payment rates to such an extraordinary degree that it would require major budgetary outlays to bring physician payment under Medicaid up to a par with that of Medicare or privately insured patients. This affects access of Medicaid patients to quality health care. Until the early 1980s both Medicare and Medicaid paid hospitals at a rate that covered their costs and was reasonably comparable with payment received from privately insured patients. Since 1981 states have been free to adopt their own Medicaid hospital payment policy, and most states have adopted more stringent reimbursement methods and levels. Medicare adopted a prospective payment system for hospitals in 1983. Since then political pressures have held increases in Medicare hospital payment rates to a very low rate. Over several years a considerable differential could be formed between the compensation rates that hospitals receive from Medicaid and Medicare and those they receive from privately insured patients. If so, it could lead to discrimination against Medicare and Medicaid patients, but it would prove costly in terms of budgetary outlays to bring Medicare and Medicaid payment rates up to a par with those of private patients.

The pluralistic, mixed public-private nature of health care financing and payment policy is deeply ingrained in the United States and seems likely to persist. Given this constraint, the most effective strategy may be to try to achieve greater coordination and integration of provider payment policy across public and private payers.

What Works to Contain Costs?

Provider payment reform initiatives have differed with respect to several characteristics: time-limited versus permanent, applicable to all patients versus to one or more subsets (such as the elderly and the disabled), state versus nationwide application, and applicable to hospitals only versus applicable to all types of health care providers. The Nixon Economic Stabilization Program was temporary, applied to all patients nationwide, and applied to all types of health care providers. State rate-setting initiatives are permanent (subject to the vagaries of the political process), typically apply to all patients but only for inpatient care, and are statewide in scope. The Carter hospital cost containment bill attempted to apply permanent controls on hospital payments for all patients nationwide. Medicare hospital prospective payment and state Medicaid hospital payment initiatives apply to subsets of patients and are permanent in nature, with Medicare extending nationwide and Medicaid initiatives typically implemented on a statewide basis. Intervening periods have been characterized as laissez-faire, with market determination of prices. The early 1980s was a period of some foment in the health care marketplace with the growth of HMOs and PPOs and a wide variety of cost containment initiatives adopted by employer health benefit plans. The general policy approach was to encourage greater consumer choice and competition among alternative types of health care providers. What has not been tried is nationwide provider payment reform applying to all patients on a permanent basis.

With respect to the initiatives that have been tried, the statistical evidence on effectiveness in containing costs is clear. Total hospital costs increased at a significantly slower rate during the Nixon Economic Stabilization Program, consideration of the Carter hospital cost containment bill, and in the first year of the Medicare PPS. Periods of freely functioning market forces were characterized by rapid rates of increase in health care costs. State rate-setting programs have slowed the rate of increase in hospital costs by about 3 percent annually.

Hospital costs per admission increased significantly more slowly under the Nixon Economic Stabilization Program, the Carter bill, the Medicare PPS, and state rate setting. Hospital costs per patient day, on the other hand, continued to increase relatively rapidly under the Medicare PPS but fared well under the other cost containment initiatives.

The Medicare prospective payment initiative has been in operation only a relatively short period of time, and its immediate impact may not be sustained over the longer term. During the first full year that it was in effect, total hospital costs and hospital costs per admission experienced a dramatic slowdown, increasing in real terms by 1.5 percent and 3.0 percent, respectively. Increases in hospital costs per patient day, on the other hand, continued to increase at historically high rates. Total health spending, including spending on nonhospital services, continued at a historically high rate in 1984 and 1985. The main effect of the Medicare PPS appears to have been shorter hospital stays for the elderly, but it is unlikely that the length of hospital stays will continue to decline in the future. The success of the Medicare PPS may well be short-term, with hospital costs returning to historical rates of increase once utilization savings have been realized. On balance it seems unlikely that the hospital cost problem has been solved on a permanent basis, and other measures may be needed in the future.

State rate-setting programs applying to all hospital patients on a permanent basis have been quite effective in restraining cost increases. States with rate-setting programs have averaged annual increases in hospital costs 3 percent lower than those in states without such programs. Over a ten-year period this differential cost performance has had an important cumulative effect. By 1984 hospital costs per capita would have been at least 87 percent higher in states with rate-setting policies had such policies not been in effect. Hospitals in states with all-payer mandatory programs have examined studies demonstrating that such programs save the Medicare program more money than the Medicare PPS would. In addition, the programs save Medicaid and privately insured patients considerable amounts. Put differently, hospitals would be making more money on Medicare patients and on other patients under the Medicare PPS than under the rate-setting systems. The success of these programs has made them politically vulnerable. Hospitals have mounted political pressure to eliminate state rate-setting programs, which cover all patients, in order to come under the Medicare PPS, which applies only to the elderly and the disabled.

Medicaid is an example of a cost containment initiative that has been effective at containing costs, but at the expense of other objectives, such as assuring access to quality health care for the poor and assuring patients the opportunity to choose their own physician. Medicaid has lowered hospital payment rates to below the rate paid by Medicare and considerably below the rate hospitals receive for the care of privately insured patients. As a result, admissions of Medicaid patients to hospitals have been declining. Further, initiatives to force all Medicaid patients to enroll in HMOs have led to abuses, inadequate care, and major disruption of care patterns for many poor. Two policy actions would help to reverse these trends: restoring Medicaid payment rates to the same level as Medicare's; and requiring states to assure Medicaid beneficiaries the freedom to choose their own health care provider, in either the HMO or the FFS sector.

Employer plans appear to have contributed to falling hospital admissions for workers and their dependents. Increased patient cost sharing and direct measures to curb hospital utilization undoubtedly account for much of this downward trend. However, these are one-time reductions in utilization. In future years hospital costs can be expected to increase at historical rates. Increased patient cost sharing shifts the financial burden of higher health care costs onto workers and their families, which is unacceptable to them in the long term and has limited potential as a future long-term strategy.

HMOs have grown markedly in the last ten years; they now enroll 8 percent of the U.S. population. HMOs tend to grow most rapidly in geographic areas with high population mobility, young families, and weak ties between patients and physicians. Given numerous barriers to HMO growth, it seems unlikely that more than one-fourth of the population will choose to receive their care from HMOs.

Evidence indicates that HMOs have lower costs than those for care rendered in the FFS sector. While HMOs have lower costs than traditional alternatives, the rate of increase in HMO costs per person are quite similar to trends over time in the FFS sector. Therefore, it seems that HMOs may be more capable of achieving a one-time downward shift in costs than of achieving a sustained slowing of costs.

The HMO model also creates a potential for underservice, since HMOs are paid the same rate regardless of how much care an individual patient receives. Patient care abuses have occurred in HMO settings, and the potential for diminished quality of care in HMOs is a genuine concern, particularly in the face of dramatic growth of for-profit owned HMOs. Federal qualification of HMOs and the establishment of stronger performance standards should help not only to reduce HMO abuses and financial failures but also to provide some assurance of quality.

PPOs are a relatively new entrant into the health care delivery system. At this point there is no evidence on the cost-effectiveness of this method of financing health care. PPOs may simply redistribute the health care cost burden among payers, reducing the cross-subsidization that currently shifts part of the cost of indigent care and medical education to privately insured patients. Without private financial support for indigent care and medical education, this financial burden will be shifted to the public sector or these important activities will be sharply curtailed. PPOs have considerable appeal to employers, however, because they encourage employees to use lower-cost hospitals and physicians. Federal qualification of PPOs might help assure the quality of providers included in such plans and protect against unsound financial practices.

There is little evidence that other cost containment initiatives have been effective. Health planning initiatives do not appear to have had much effect on health care costs, perhaps because of the absence of genuine incentives on the part of planning agencies to disapprove proposed projects. Utilization review and quality assurance initiatives, such as PSROs and their successors, PROs, appear to be marginally effective. PRO activities under Medicare may deserve credit for keeping hospital admissions down under PPS, which otherwise gives hospitals an incentive to increase admissions of the elderly. Voluntary efforts by the hospital industry to control costs have not proven effective in the absence of genuine threats of mandatory controls.

Doing nothing has been the least effective approach to containing health care costs. The health sector has exhibited a strong and persistent tendency to outstrip the rest of the economy in growing expenditures except during periods of direct intervention to contain cost increases. The health care cost problem will neither solve itself nor be easily solved. However, the many initiatives that have been instituted do provide valuable lessons and point the way toward an effective long-term policy toward limiting increases in health care costs.

Other Impacts

It is considerably easier to assess the effectiveness of health care cost containment initiatives in curbing the increase in costs than in achieving more basic policy goals. Obviously, the goal is not to lower costs but to improve productive efficiency (resulting in the provision of health care services at a lower cost) or allocative efficiency (resulting in provision of only those health care services that significantly benefit patients). To the extent that health care costs are rising at a slower rate because the poor are being squeezed out of the health care system, the elderly are being discharged prematurely from hospitals, or needed care is being postponed, social goals are not being met. In practice, various cost containment initiatives that are effective in containing costs probably achieve a mix of outcomes—some improvements in efficiency and some loss in medically important health care services for some population groups.

There is considerable evidence that cost containment initiatives, especially those instituted under Medicaid, are having the effect of reducing health care to the poor. Increasing numbers of people have no health insurance, in part because of cutbacks in Medicaid and in part because of a reduction in employer-based health coverage. Transfers of patients without health insurance are up, as patients are turned away from for-profit and private nonprofit hospitals because of an inability to pay their bills. For the poor covered by Medicaid, restrictive hospital payment policies are reducing the attractiveness of Medicaid patients to hospitals and leading to a reduction in hospital care for Medicaid patients. Curtailment in Medicaid payments and the growth of PPO plans have put greater pressure on teaching hospitals, which provide much of the care to the poor, and could lead to further reductions in access to care of the poor in the future.

Increased cost sharing under employer plans and under Medicare have shifted some of the financial burden for health care onto patients, many of whom have relatively modest incomes. Earlier hospital discharges have also increased financial burdens on the elderly and disabled, as prescription drugs and many other health care services needed during recuperation are not covered or are covered on a less extensive basis once the patient is discharged from the hospital.

Biomedical research and graduate medical education are also likely to be adversely affected by cost containment initiatives. Growth of PPOs and HMOs channel patients away from expensive teaching hospitals, thus reducing the cross-subsidization of teaching and research from patient care revenues. The Medicare PPS is also likely to place tighter restrictions on payments to teaching hospitals in the future, which will in turn further erode support for research and medical education. To date these activities have been protected by generous allowances for teaching hospitals in the Medicare PPS. If PPS payment rates increase more slowly than the rate of inflation, some deterioration in innovative biomedical research and medical education seems inevitable unless other sources of support for them are found.

Cost containment initiatives all have the potential to reduce the quality of care provided to patients. Most of these initiatives have been imposed on a health care system with considerable inefficiency and slack. As incentives to reduce cost are created, some waste and inefficiency can be readily identified and eliminated. It is difficult to be sanguine, however, about the potential for future savings to come without any loss in quality of care. Nor do good systems exist to monitor changes in quality and to inform patients of the implications for patient care of the new incentives being put in place. Much more research is needed to evaluate the impacts of alternative cost containment initiatives on the quality of patient care.

Major Concerns

Experience with public sector and private sector health care cost containment initiatives provides many lessons on which to draw in designing future policy options. This experience leaves many concerns unresolved, however, and clearly suggests that future action will be needed to mount effective cost containment measures and to remedy some of the undesired side effects of such measures. In summary, the major concerns to be addressed by future policy action include the following:

- The health care cost problem has not been solved but has hit a period of temporary respite through one-time savings from reduced utilization of hospital services.
- There are still productivity and efficiency gains to be made in the health sector.
- Cost containment initiatives instituted to date have had a serious adverse effect on the nation's poor and have increased the financial burdens placed on the elderly, the disabled, and workers and their families.
- Teaching hospitals are likely to come under severe financial pressures in the future, leading to a reduction in care for the indigent, biomedical research, and medical education.
- Cost containment initiatives have the potential to slow the rate of technological progress in the health sector and lead to a deterioration

in the quality of care. No effective monitoring systems exist to detect such changes and to alert patients and policy makers about them.

- Budgetary pressures on federal and state governments could widen the gap between payment rates for patients covered under public programs and those for patients covered by private health insurance plans. Such a differential has the potential to undermine the quality and accessibility of care for the most vulnerable members of society and will be increasingly difficult to remedy.

- The focus on cost reduction to the exclusion of other important social goals is likely to lead to an unbalanced policy agenda with inadequate attention being given to guaranteeing access to quality health care.

Chapter 12

**Future Directions for the U.S.
Health Care System: A Long-Range
Policy Proposal**

With few exceptions, efforts to contain health care costs have been
fragmented and their effectiveness has been limited. In large part this
reflects the structure of the U.S. health care financing system, with Medicare, Medicaid, and employer-provided health insurance each independently pursuing cost containment policies developed with their own interests in mind. This approach to cost containment has not succeeded in
controlling health care costs. In addition, those suffering the brunt of this
uncoordinated policy have been the uninsured and the poor, who have
been discriminated against by a market-oriented health system.

Cost containment by insurers must be integrated into a unified policy
in order to be effective. In addition, cost containment initiatives must be
considered as part of a broader array of social goals—goals related to
improving and maintaining the health of the public, access to care, quality
of care, and commitment to excellence in research and technology. The
following section sets forth a set of goals that should guide health care
policy in the future. This is followed by a long-range policy proposal
aimed at meeting multiple objectives for the health care system. This plan
could be phased in over time as budget resources permit and as experience
with each step is gained.

The primary advantage of an incremental approach is its adaptability
to changing conditions in both the public and the private sector. It is
especially well suited to the federal budget process, which constantly
weighs competing budget priorities. New initiatives are feasible in a tight
budget framework, but only if they are relatively modest in scope. Current
programs are familiar to legislators, fall within clearly defined jurisdic-
tional boundaries, and have advocates among members of authorizing
committees. New programs, particularly those that are sweeping in nature, are too filled with uncertainty to prompt action on a tight legislative
calendar.

There is, of course, a down side to an incremental approach. More attractive elements of a long-term package may be enacted first, leaving no momentum for further change. Administrative systems that maintain multiple programs may be more complex than a newly designed system. Tight cost control measures may also be more difficult to coordinate among multiple programs, which can be played off against each other by providers.

Goals for the U.S. Health Care System

In a world of constrained resources, tradeoffs must be made among multiple goals. Resources for health care could alternatively be used to improve education, clean up our harbors, invest in major scientific research endeavors, or modernize the industrial plant and equipment. Workers who are busy building hospitals or health centers could be building roads or repairing bridges. Young people could be attracted into careers in science and engineering or education rather than nursing and medicine. As a society, we need to pose questions about whether we would be better off with a higher or lower share of our nation's resources going into the health sector.

Even if improving and maintaining the population's health is viewed as a top priority and worthy of considerable resources, questions need to be raised about whether further investment in the health care sector yields the highest payoff in terms of improved health. Alternatively, the standard of living of the poor could be improved, resources could be invested in ensuring that everyone has an adequate diet, and housing, workplaces, and communities could be made safer and healthier places in which to live, work, and play. These uses of economic resources should be weighed against spending on hospital, physician, and other health care services.

Improving performance within the health care sector to achieve greater value in terms of health outcomes for the resources devoted to health care is an important overall goal. It should be recognized, however, that the pursuit of improved efficiency may sometimes conflict with the pursuit of improved health outcomes. A desire to control costs may compromise the goal of improving access to and quality of care. Acceptability and freedom to choose among alternatives may also be in conflict with goals of limiting costs. Consequently, it is necessary to explicate those goals that most Americans value most highly and to evaluate the impact of alternative policy directions on those goals. As a starting point for such a process, we propose the following seven goals.

Goal 1. Reduce preventable mortality and morbidity. The World Health Organization (WHO) has urged the adoption of "Health for All by the Year 2000" as a major goal of all countries. This goal calls for achieving the maximum attainable health and social well-being of the population. The United States, along with nations around the world, has committed itself to achieving major improvements in the health of the population by the end of the century. The U.S. commitment was embodied in the report of the Surgeon General entitled *Healthy People* and renewed in presentations before the World Health Assembly. In response to the WHO initiative, the United States has established goals of reducing preventable mortality and morbidity by establishing a set of health objectives to be achieved through improvements in lifestyles, reduction in occupational and environmental hazards, and accessibility of preventive health care services to the entire population.

Goal 2. Enhance the quality of life of all individuals by maintaining their functional capacity as long as possible and by relieving avoidable pain and discomfort. As the population of the United States ages, more attention is being given to the quality of life at the end of the life span. Some health conditions are terminal in nature and require primarily hospice care to relieve pain and assist the individual and his or her family in making the most of the time remaining. Other chronic conditions, such as Alzheimer's disease, lead to a slow deterioration in mental or physical functioning. For such conditions the primary goal should be to maintain functioning capacity as long as possible, to provide support for the patient and family, and to guarantee the patient and family control over major decisions affecting the nature of care (e.g., whether or not the patient should be placed in a nursing home or receive high-technology care).

Goal 3. Assure that no one is denied health care because of an inability to pay. One of the most important social goals we should try to achieve is to assure access to adequate health care services for the entire population. This is of particular importance for the most vulnerable members of society. The poor, for example, are unable to afford costly health care without assistance. An optimal health care system would assure that no one is turned away from care because of inability to pay or complex needs.

Goal 4. Assure that the financial burden of health care expenses is equitably distributed. No one should be required to pay health bills that are high in relation to his or her family financial resources. Catastrophic illness can pose a hardship for nearly everyone; even minor illnesses or accidents can result in serious financial hardship to the uninsured poor.

Goal 5. Promote efficiency and effectiveness in the provision of health care services. Despite the high expectations that Americans have for their health sector, they are also concerned with high outlays for health care. They would like to improve productivity and efficiency in the health sector by eliminating waste or unnecessary services and assuring that health benefits are received in proportion to money spent on health care. This requires a health systems approach to health care delivery.

Goal 6. Preserve or enhance the quality of health care. Americans have come to expect and demand high-quality health care. They expect their physicians to be dedicated, well trained, and highly qualified and to recommend a course of diagnosis and treatment that is in the patient's best interest. They expect hospitals and other health care facilities to be adequately equipped and staffed with qualified trained personnel and to be committed to the delivery of appropriate care. Americans also desire continued technological progress and breakthroughs in biomedical research.

Goal 7. Maintain the right of individuals to make choices individually or collectively through a democratic political process. Individual rights are an integral part of American culture. Americans expect to be informed about choices affecting their lives and well-being and to have a say in those decisions. They feel strongly about the right to choose their own physician or health delivery system and to vote with their feet if they are dissatisfied with the care or advice they receive. Just as individuals want the right to make individual choices, they expect the right to make some decisions on a collective basis through a democratic political process.

Choosing among Alternatives

Clearly, it is unrealistic to expect to achieve all of these social goals. Therefore, a mechanism needs to be devised to evaluate policy alternatives with these social goals in mind and to resolve inherent conflicts between individual goals. While different individuals may weigh the importance of these goals differently, a thorough analysis of policy options should define the impact of the options on access, equity, health, quality of life, quality of care, progress, and free choice, as well as the implications for the cost of care and its distribution among alternative sources of financing. In addition, policy alternatives should be evaluated in terms of the following criteria.

Effectiveness in containing costs. Any policy proposal should be evaluated with a clear understanding of its costs, including additional real economic resources that must be diverted to the health sector and the budgetary costs to different levels of government. Estimates should also be available on costs shifted from the public sector to the private sector, or the reverse, and any change in cost to different individuals. Estimates of economic and budgetary costs should be available both for the point of implementation and over time.

Acceptability. Policy options must be acceptable to patients, health care providers, and those who pay for health care services received by others. If policy options are to be viable in the long term, they need to correspond with patient expectations. The initiatives need to be simple enough to be easily understood. Similarly, physicians and other health care providers need to find policy options that are acceptable in order to avoid mass opposition or boycotting of a program.

Administrative feasibility. Any policy option should be relatively easy to administer. Simplicity is desirable, both for ease of understanding and for administrative purposes.

Political feasibility. Finally, policy options need to be able to elicit political support from major interest groups—labor, business, insurance, physicians, hospitals, and consumer groups such as senior citizens' organizations and advocacy groups. Political support from all geographical regions is important, as is support from state and local government officials. While a consensus of all parties is extraordinarily difficult to obtain, accommodation to major concerns can help mitigate opposition.

A Long-Range Policy Proposal

The long-range policy proposal presented here is concerned equally with assuring health insurance coverage of the entire population and containing health care costs. It has two major components: (1) universal health insurance coverage; and (2) reform of the health care system through greater coordination and equalization of provider payment among Medicare, Medicaid, and private insurance plans and greater emphasis on incentives for efficiency through promotion of HMOs.

Health Care Insurance Coverage

The central element of the long-range policy proposal is universal health insurance coverage through expansions in coverage under existing public and private health insurance plans. This coverage may be obtained through different approaches. The first approach is to require employers to cover employees and their dependents through private group health insurance plans. The second approach involves greater incentives for the purchase of private health insurance, such as eliminating excessive mandated requirements, encouraging the establishment of insurance pools with broadly based financing, including contributions by self-insured employers, and provision of vouchers to permit the uninsured to purchase private health insurance. The third approach involves public programs that would, for example, cover all elderly and disabled under Medicare, cover all poor under Medicaid, and give any otherwise uninsured person the option of buying Medicaid coverage or coverage from an insurance pool on a sliding-scale contributory basis. Given political and economic constraints, a mixed public-private approach with a combination of these options is probably the most viable. These options could be designed as follows.

Option 1. Employer Mandate

Coverage of all full-time workers and their dependents under employer health plans could be required by law, and minimum benefit standards would be prescribed. Standards could apply to all firms, whether they elected to self-insure or to purchase coverage through health insurers. Specific elements include the following:

Eligibility. Employers would be required to cover all their full-time employees, as well as the employees' spouses and dependents. No worker or dependent could be denied coverage, nor could preexisting conditions be excluded from coverage.

Extension of coverage. Coverage would begin upon employment and would continue at least ninety days after termination of employment, or after the death of a worker or divorce of a worker and spouse. During this postemployment period the employer would continue to share in the premium cost. Employees and their dependents would be given the right to continue coverage at group rates after this period for as long as they chose to pay the full group premium cost plus an administrative fee.

Benefits. The minimum benefit package would include inpatient hospital services, physician services, and prenatal, delivery, and infant care. Employers could provide a broader benefit package, but not less than the minimum.

Catastrophic coverage. Proposed employer plans could include patient deductibles and coinsurance (with the exception of maternal and infant care), but cost sharing for a family would be subject to a ceiling not exceeding a certain level. Annual deductibles and coinsurance rates would be limited.

Choice of an HMO or PPO. All qualified employer plans would be required to give employees and their dependents a choice of enrollment in any federally qualified HMO or other case-managed approaches, such as PPOs, when those are available in the community, elect to be offered, and are administratively feasible for employers to provide.

Financing. Employers would be required to pay a specific percentage of premium costs for the mandated plan. Higher employer premium shares could, of course, be provided. Today, more than 85 percent of workers with employer-financed insurance are covered by plans in which the employer pays at least 75 percent of the premium. Any employer whose premium contribution for a minimum plan exceeds 5 percent of payroll would be eligible to purchase Medicaid coverage for the minimum benefit package at a premium contribution not to exceed 5 percent of payroll.

Administration. Employer plans would be federally qualified. Penalties would be assessed for misrepresentation or nonconformance with federal standards.

Reinsurance. Employer plans, HMOs, and PPOs would be eligible to buy reinsurance protection against the costs of truly extraordinary illness (over $25,000 per covered person) through private insurance companies.

Option 2. Incentives for Private Health Insurance

Individuals would be encouraged to purchase health insurance from private insurance companies. Excessive regulatory requirements, which now make private insurance too costly, would need to be eliminated, and better tax incentives or other forms of financing would be necessary to expand coverage of the uninsured. Specific elements of this approach include the following:

• Elimination of state-mandated health benefits

• Establishment of state risk pools with broadly based financing, including contributions from self-insured employers

• One hundred percent tax deductibility of health insurance premiums for the self-employed

• Vouchers for the purchase of private health insurance subsidized by state or federal tax revenues

Under the voucher plan, premiums would be subsidized for low-income persons, and changes in the tax code would be used to finance a part of the cost. Specifically, the approach would include the following provisions:

Eligibility. Participants would be expected to purchase health insurance through the private insurance sector.

Benefits. A minimum benefits package would be established by federal legislation. It would include specific benefits such as inpatient hospital services, physician services, and prenatal, delivery, and infant care or the actuarial equivalent.

Choice of an HMO or PPO. Participants would have the options of using vouchers to enroll in an HMO or PPO.

Financing. Participants would receive a tax rebate for health insurance. Rebates for singles and families would differ but would not be tied to income or how tax deductions are calculated. Participants with an income below a certain threshold would receive a federal subsidy to purchase health insurance.

Administration. The program would be administered by the federal government. Minimum benefits would be assigned by the Department of Health and Human Services, and compliance would be monitored by the Internal Revenue Service. States would ensure that public and private insurance options were available to their residents.

Reinsurance. Insurers could reinsure.

Option 3. Medicaid

The Medicaid program would be expanded to provide acute health care benefits to the entire population falling outside employer-mandated coverage and Medicare coverage. Medicaid would be a secondary payer for individuals covered under employer plans or Medicare.

Eligibility. All individuals whose income fell below the federal poverty level could be automatically covered under Medicaid. Coverage would be independent of assets. Categorical restrictions would be removed so that single individuals and childless couples would be covered. Medicaid acute-care benefits would also be available to others not eligible for coverage under employer plans in exchange for a premium set on a sliding scale with income. The premium would range from zero for those below the federal poverty level to 100 percent of the actuarial value of the Medicaid acute-care benefit package for those with incomes more than twice the federal poverty level.

Benefits. The Medicaid program would cover the current acute-care mandatory benefits plus prescription drugs, without arbitrary limits on amount, duration, or scope of benefits. Unnecessary use of services would be discouraged through utilization review and prior authorization provisions. For individuals purchasing coverage with a sliding-scale premium, modest cost-sharing provisions could be included. Health care providers would be paid at a level comparable to that under Medicare.

Financing and administration. The net new costs of expanded Medicaid coverage would be met through federal general revenues. States, however, could continue to contribute a uniform, but lower, matching rate for all Medicaid beneficiaries. Administration of coverage for new beneficiaries would be handled through state Medicaid administrative procedures.

Health System Reform

The second portion of the proposed plan involves changing the methods of paying hospitals, physicians, and HMOs and implementing other measures to promote enrollment in HMOs and PPOs.

Provider Payment Reform

Major reforms in current methods of paying hospitals, physicians, and HMOs would be implemented. Medicaid payment rules would follow those of Medicare, with state waivers for states that can meet performance criteria, including comparability between levels of Medicare and Medicaid payment. Employer plans would follow Medicare payment principles or an approved alternative that meets comparability criteria.

Hospitals. The DRG PPS for hospitals under Medicare would be retained and improved. Major modifications in the current system would include:

- A formula for establishing increases in PPS rates or establishment of three-year rates of increase by statute
- Incorporating an adjustment in payment rates based on the severity of cases in order to reimburse hospitals more appropriately for very expensive patients
- Refinements to the method of financing medical education, biomedical research, and technology diffusion
- Incorporating an additional percentage allowance in the DRG payment rate to cover the cost of capital
- Encouraging states to institute or maintain their own all-payer hospital prospective payment systems, meeting the tests of generating at least the same level of budgetary savings as the DRG PPS and assuring equity among payers
- Medicare hospital payment provisions for Medicaid, with the relative DRG prospective payment rates and levels adjusted to reflect the resource cost of caring for the nonelderly Medicaid population

Physicians. Physicians would be paid according to a fee schedule under Medicare and Medicaid. The determination of a method of establishing relative values should be postponed pending further research and analysis of alternatives. The level of the fee schedule would be set to achieve approximately the same level of public expenditure as would be achieved without the change; that is, it would generate neither budgetary savings nor costs. Annual increases in the fee schedule would be pegged to achieve increases in total physician expenditures no greater than preset targets.

HMOs

Medicare, Medicaid, and employer plans would be encouraged to offer enrollees a choice of federally qualified HMOs if they are locally available. Federal qualification standards would be strengthened and closely monitored to ensure quality of care and fiscal soundness. Specific requirements include:

- Freedom of choice between health services provided on a fee-for-service basis and HMOs for all Medicare and Medicaid beneficiaries
- Multiple capitated plans wherever possible, with no more than half of the enrollees in any plan drawn from a single payer source
- A minimum benefit package including the services required in the employer minimum health benefit plans
- That all HMOs and insurance plans offer an open enrollment periods
- Clear, objective, and comprehensive information on the various options to be provided by employers, unions, government, or whoever is providing services
- That HMO capitation payment rates be derived from anticipated health expenditures based on enrollee health status, but premiums paid by enrollees must not vary with health status
- Federal certification of HMOs based on quality of care and financial soundness criteria

Evaluation of the Proposal

This plan has several key characteristics:

- It is designed to make major gains in the achievement of the goals set forth above.
- It is a pluralistic plan with opportunities for the federal government, states, and the private sector to design health plans meeting their own special needs.
- It is incremental in nature but presents a vision of the ultimately desired system.
- It assumes that implementation of the long-range policy proposal will be achieved in phases over time rather than through a single legislative measure.

The criteria of administrative and political feasibility, in particular, rule out the wholesale adoption of health financing systems from other countries in favor of a mixed public-private system. It assumes that health care services in the United States will continue to be provided predominantly by private nonprofit or for-profit organizations and that patients will continue to have the option of selecting from a mix of FFS and prepaid modes of practice.

This proposal primarily emphasizes reform of health care financing, including health insurance coverage for all; coordinated methods of paying physicians, hospitals, and other health care providers; and incentives to reform the organization and delivery of health care services to promote efficiency and quality of care.

The proposal would contribute to improving the health of the population by removing financial barriers to medical care and increasing funding for prevention and primary care. Maternity and infant care services would be covered without cost sharing for those covered by both employer plans and Medicaid. Improved access to acute care for the uninsured would improve health and give children a better chance for a productive life.

Universal access to health care services would be guaranteed through coverage of the entire population under employer health plans, other private health insurance plans or pools, Medicare, or Medicaid. Employer plans, HMOs, and PPOs would not be permitted to exclude high-risk individuals or to charge them higher premiums.

The proposal would lead to a more equitable distribution of the financial burden of health care expenses. Maximum out-of-pocket ceilings on health care expenses would be instituted in all plans. Incentives to control costs and improve efficiency would be provided through numerous provider payment and system reform provisions. Quality standards would be developed and monitored through Medicare, Medicaid, HMOs, and PPOs. Provider payment rates would be set to ensure continued room for technological progress and development. Individuals would be given information and choices among alternative health plans.

Precise cost estimates of the long-range proposal are not now available. Cost estimates of proposals for mandating universal health insurance coverage under all three options would depend upon the specific features of each proposal. Mandating employer health insurance coverage is likely to cost employers on the order of $25–35 billion in 1990, depending on the benefit package and employer premium share. The option of encouraging the purchase of private health insurance through the provision of vouchers could cost federal or state governments $10–20 billion, depending upon the generosity of the vouchers. Federal tax relief could be generated to offset this cost by changing the tax treatment of fringe benefits. The option of expanding Medicaid coverage to the poor and subsidizing Medicaid coverage of the near-poor could cost $10–15 billion in federal and state outlays. These new public or private outlays could be offset in part by provider payment reform and incentives for improved efficiency in the health care system.

The long-range policy proposal builds on current programs and continues current administrative mechanisms. For example, state agencies would continue to have responsibility for enrolling the poor in Medicaid. Policy regarding provider payment would be established by intermediaries under Medicare. Some new administrative mechanisms would need to be established, however, to monitor the quality of care and fiscal soundness of a greater variety of health plans. More individuals would become eligible under Medicaid, and many smaller employers would be required to provide health insurance to workers and dependents for the first time.

The long-range policy proposal can be expected to have significant political support and opposition. It would ensure new revenues for the health sector through expanded insurance coverage. This should prove attractive to the hospital sector and certain groups of physicians, especially newly trained physicians. Primary care physicians should welcome the new physician payment reform; but it could prove threatening to surgeons and other specialty physicians, depending on how relative values are established. It should receive support from consumer groups and labor. Small businesses may be concerned by the new proposed administrative and financial burdens. The insurance industry should be supportive of those approaches that expand employer-based coverage and yet preserve a role for small group and individual health insurance coverage, while leaving primary responsibility for coverage of the poor and near-poor to an expanded Medicaid program. Recognition of the problems of the uninsured, poor children and women, and the low-income elderly is growing and should increase broad public support; however, substantial federal budget deficits limit the political feasibility of any approach that requires major increases in government outlays.

The political feasibility of the proposal could be improved by a phased implementation. Modest incremental improvements in public programs and private insurance plans could be made. Experience with these changes could be obtained before moving on to the next phase. For example, it is possible to begin by expanding Medicaid coverage for those with an income below 75 percent of the poverty level, then to expand coverage for those with an income below 100 percent of the poverty level, and then to relax the assets test. Employer plan standards could first be applied to larger firms or modified with smaller employer premium contributions. Provider payment reform provisions could be phased in gradually, gaining experience with each successive round of legislation. It is extremely desirable, however, that such a phased-in approach move each component of the proposal forward in each phase. Otherwise politically popular elements will be enacted first and no action will be taken on the more controversial elements.

A long-range policy proposal, regardless of its ultimate shape, would greatly improve the health policy deliberation process. The current system of relying on year-to-year changes in health financing programs without any consensus on a longer-range plan leads to gimmickry and instability in the health system. It gives undue weight to the fiscal objective of cutting budgetary outlays instead of basing health policy on social goals to be achieved by the health sector. It is hoped that this long-range policy proposal will facilitate informed debate leading to such a consensus.

References

Aaron, H. J. 1984. "Alternative Medicare Financing Sources." *Milbank Memorial Fund Quarterly* 62, no. 2:349–55.

Abernethy, D. S., and D. A. Pearson. 1979. *Regulating Hospital Costs: The Development of Public Policy.* Ann Arbor, Mich.: AUPHA Press.

Abramowitz, M. 1986. "Workers Share More of Health Care Burden." *Washington Post,* 7 July, Washington Business, p. 1.

Alex Brown & Sons, Inc. 1984. *The HMO Industry: A Marketing Research Report.* Baltimore: Health Care Stocks Department, January.

———. 1986. *Health Maintenance Organization Industry Trends.* Baltimore: Health Care Group, December.

Altman, D., R. Greene, and H. Sapolsky. 1981. *Health Planning and Regulation: The Decision-making Process.* Ann Arbor, Mich.: AUPHA Press.

Altman, S. H., and J. Eichenholz. 1976. "Inflation in the Health Industry: Causes and Cures." In *Health: A Victim or Cause of Inflation?* edited by Michael Zubkoff, pp. 7–30. New York: Milbank Memorial Fund.

American Hospital Association (AHA). 1982. *Health Care: What Happens to People When Government Cuts Back.* Report of the Special Committee on Federal Funding of Mental Health and Other Services. Chicago, 13 August.

———. 1985. *Hospital Statistics, 1985 edition.* Chicago.

———. 1986. *Hospital Statistics, 1986 edition.* Chicago.

———. 1987. *Hospital Statistics, 1987 edition.* Chicago.

———. 1988. *Hospital Statistics, 1988 edition.* Chicago.

American Medical Association (AMA). 1985. "American Medical Association DRG Monitoring Project." Report to the AMA, House of Delegates. December.

American Medical Care Review Association (AMCRA). 1986. *Directory of Preferred Provider Organizations and the Industry Report on PPO Development.* Bethesda, Md.

American Medical Peer Review Association (AMPRA). 1985. "PROs: The Future Agenda." A Report of the American Medical Peer Review Association's Task Force on PRO Implementation. September.

American Society of Internal Medicine. 1985. "The Impacts of DRGs in Patient Care." *American Society of Internal Medicine Newsletter.* October.

Anderson, G. F. 1986. "Prospective Payment for Capital." Testimony before the Senate Finance Committee, 14 March. Washington, D.C.: GPO.

Anderson, G. F., J. C. Cantor, E. P. Steinberg, and J. Holloway. 1986a. "Capitation Pricing: Adjusting for Prior Utilization and Physician Discretion." *Health Care Financing Review* 8, no. 2:27–34.

———. 1986b. "Paying for HMO Care: Issues in Setting Capitation Rates." *Milbank Memorial Fund Quarterly* 64, no. 4:548–65.

Anderson, G. F., and J. E. Erickson. 1986. "DataWatch: National Medical Care Spending." *Health Affairs* 5 (Fall): 96–104.

Anderson, G. F., and P. Ginsburg. 1983. "Prospective Capital Payments to Hospitals." *Health Affairs* 2 (Fall): 52–53.

———. 1984. "Medicare Payment and Hospital Capital: Future Policy Options." *Health Affairs* 3 (Fall): 35–48.

Anderson, G. F., and J. Knickman. 1984. "Patterns of Expenditure among High Utilizers of Medical Care Services: The Experience of Medicare Beneficiaries from 1974 to 1977." *Medical Care* 22, no. 2:143–49.

Anderson, G. F., and J. Lave. 1986. "Financing Graduate Medical Education Using Multiple Regression to Set Payment Rates." *Inquiry* 23, no. 2:191–99.

Anderson, G. F., and E. P. Steinberg. 1984a. "Hospital Readmissions of the Medicare Population." *New England Journal of Medicine* 311, no. 21:1344–53.

———. 1984b. "To Buy or Not to Buy: Technology Acquisition under Prospective Payment." *New England Journal of Medicine* 311, no. 3:182–85.

———. 1986. "DRGs and Specialized Nutrition Support: The Need for Reform." *Journal of Parenteral and Enteral Nutrition* 10, no. 1:3–8.

Anderson, M. D., and P. Fox. 1987. "Lessons from Medicaid Managed Care." *Health Affairs* 6 (Spring): 71–86.

Arnould, R. J., L. W. Debrock, and J. W. Pollard. 1984. "Do HMOs Provide Specific Services More Efficiently?" *Inquiry* 21, no. 3:243–53.

Arthur D. Little, Inc. 1985. "The Health Care System in the Mid 1990s." *Modern Healthcare* 15 (5 July): 22.

Arthur Young. 1986. *Financing of Graduate Medical Education*. Final Report submitted to the Assistant Secretary for Planning and Evaluation, U.S. Department of Health and Human Services. Washington, D.C.

A. S. Hansen, Inc. 1985. "Hansen Survey of Medical Plans and Practices." Deerfield, Ill.

Ashby, J. L. 1984. *The Inequity of Medicare Prospective Payment in Large Urban Areas.* Washington, D.C.: District of Columbia Hospital Association, September.

Bauer, K. 1977. "Ratesetting—This Way to Salvation?" *Milbank Memorial Fund Quarterly* 55, no. 1:117–58.

Beebe, S., J. Lubitz, and P. Eggers. 1985. "Using Prior Utilization to Determine Payments for Medicare Enrollees in Health Maintenance Organizations." *Health Care Financing Review* 6, no. 3:27–36.

Berki, S. E., and M. Ashcraft. 1980. "HMO Enrollment: Who Joins What and Why—A Review of the Literature." *Milbank Memorial Fund Quarterly* 58, no. 4:588–632.

Berman, R. 1986. "Severity of Illness and the Teaching Hospitals." *Journal of Medical Education* 61, no. 1:1–9.

Bieber, O. 1985. "Bargaining for Equitable, Cost-effective Health Care." *Business and Health* 2, no. 5:20–24.

Biles, B., C. J. Schramm, and J. G. Atkinson. 1980. "Hospital Cost Inflation under State Rate-setting Programs." *New England Journal of Medicine* 303, no. 12:664–68.

Blendon, R. J. 1986a. "Health Policy Choices for the 1990s." *Issues in Science and Technology* 2, no. 4:65–73.

———. 1986b. Presentation to the Fourth National Conference on Hospital-Medical Public Policy Issues, Washington, D.C., 18 July.

Blendon, R. J., and D. Altman. 1984. "Public Attitudes about Health-Care Costs." *New England Journal of Medicine* 311, no. 9:613–16.

Blendon, R. J., D. Altman, and S. M. Kilstein. 1983. "Health Insurance for the Unemployed and Uninsured." *National Journal* 15, no. 22:1146–49.

Blendon, R. J., and T. W. Moloney. 1982. "Perspectives on the Medicaid Crisis." In *New Approaches to the Medicaid Crisis*, edited by R. J. Blendon and T. W. Moloney, pp. 3–18. Proceedings of the 1981 Commonwealth Fund Forum. New York: F&S Press.

Blendon, R. J., and D. E. Rogers. 1983. "Cutting Medical Care Costs: *Primum Non Nocere.*" *Journal of the American Medical Association* 250, no. 14:1880–85.

Blumberg, M. S. 1980. "Health Status and Health Care Use by Type of Private Health Coverage." *Milbank Memorial Fund Quarterly* 58, no. 4:633–55.

Bovbjerg, R. R., and J. Holahan. 1982. *Medicaid in the Reagan Era: Federal Policy and State Choices.* Washington, D.C.: Urban Institute Press.

Bovbjerg, R. R., and C. Koller. 1986. "State Insurance Pools: Current Performance and Future Prospects." *Inquiry* 22, no. 2:111–21.

Brook, R. H., and K. L. Kahn. 1985. "The Impact of DRG-based Prospective Payment System (PPS) on Quality of Care for Hospitalized Medicare Patients." Proposal submitted to the Health Care Financing Administration, U.S. Department of Health and Human Services. Santa Monica: Rand Corporation.

Brook, R. H., and K. N. Lohr. 1982. "Second-Opinion Programs: Beyond Cost-benefit Analyses." *Medical Care* 20, no. 1:1–2.

Brook, R. H., K. N. Lohr, M. R. Chassin, J. Kosekoff, A. Fink, and D. H. Solomon. 1984. "Geographic Variations in the Use of Services: Do They Have Any Clinical Significance?" *Health Affairs* 3 (Summer): 63–73.

Brook, R. H., J. E. Ware, W. H. Rogers, E. B. Keeler, A. R. Davies, C. A. Donald, G. A. Goldberg, K. N. Lohr, P. C. Masthay, and J. P. Newhouse. 1983. "Does Free Care Improve Adult Health?" *New England Journal of Medicine* 309, no. 23:1426–34.

Brown, E. R., M. R. Cousineau, and W. T. Price. 1985. "Competing for Medi-Cal Business: Why Hospitals Did, and Did Not, Get Contracts." *Inquiry* 22, no. 3:237–50.

Brown, L. D. 1983. *Politics and Health Care Organization: HMOs as a Federal Policy.* Washington, D.C.: Brookings Institution.

Brown, R. 1983. "Public Hospitals on the Brink: Their Problems and Their Options." *Journal of Health Politics, Policy and Law* 7, no. 4:227–44.

Califano, J. A., Jr. 1977. Testimony before the Senate Finance Committee.

————. 1986. *America's Health Care Revolution: Who Lives? Who Dies? Who Pays?* New York: Random House.

Cameron, J. 1985. "The Indirect Costs of Graduate Medical Education." *New England Journal of Medicine* 311, no. 20:1314–17.

Carr, W. J., and P. J. Feldstein. 1967. "The Relationship of Cost to Hospital Size." *Inquiry* 4, no. 1:45–65.

Chassin, M. R. 1983. "Variations in Hospital Length of Stay: Their Relationship to Health Outcomes." Office of Technology Assessment, Health Technology Case Study No. 24. Washington, D.C.: GPO, August.

Chassin, M. R., R. H. Brook, R. E. Park, J. Keesey, A. Fink, J. Kosecoff, K. L. Kahn, N. J. Merrick, and D. H. Solomon. 1986. "Variations in the Use of Medical and Surgical Services by the Medicare Population." *New England Journal of Medicine* 314, no. 5:285–89.

Chassin, M. R., J. Kosecoff, R. E. Park, C. M. Winslow, K. L. Kahn, N. J. Merrick, J. Keesey, A. Fink, D. H. Solomon, and R. H. Brook. 1987. "Does Inappropriate Use Explain Geographic Variations in the Use of Health Care Services?" *Journal of the American Medical Association* 258, no. 18:2533–37.

Coelen, C., and D. Sullivan. 1981. "An Analysis of the Effects of Prospective Reimbursement Programs on Hospital Expenditures." *Health Care Financing Review* 2, no. 3:1–40.

Cohodes, D. 1983. "Which Will Survive? The $150 Billion Capital Question." *Inquiry* 21, no. 2:5–11.

Cohodes, D., and B. Kinkead. 1984. *Hospital Capital Formation in the 1980s.* Baltimore: Johns Hopkins University Press.

Commonwealth Fund Task Force on Academic Health Centers. 1985. *Prescription for Change: Report of the Task Force on Academic Health Centers.* New York: Commonwealth Fund.

Cromwell, J., and S. Hurdle. 1986. "National Impact Study of Alternative Reimbursement Waivers." Medicaid Program Evaluation Working Paper 3.6. Prepared for the Health Care Financing Administration, U.S. Department of Health and Human Services. Machine copy.

Cromwell, J., and J. Kanak. 1982. "The Effects of Prospective Reimbursement Programs on Hospital Adoption and Service Sharing." *Health Care Financing Review* 4, no. 2:67–88.

Cunningham, F., and J. Williamson. 1980. "How Does the Quality of Health Care in HMOs Compare to That in Other Settings?" *Group Health Journal* 1:4–25.

Dans, P. E., J. P. Weiner, and S. E. Otter. 1985. "Peer Review Organizations, Promises and Potential Pitfalls." *New England Journal of Medicine* 313, no. 18:1131–37.

Davis, C. 1986. "The Future of Prospective Payment Systems and Diagnosis-related Groups." Presentation at conference on Analysis of Recent Surgical Health Policy: Hospitals at Risk, New York, 15 May.

Davis, K. 1975. *National Health Insurance: Benefits, Costs, and Consequences.* Washington, D.C.: Brookings Institution.

———. 1981. "Recent Trends in Hospital Costs: Failure of the Voluntary Effort." Testimony before the House Committee on Energy and Commerce, 15 December. Washington, D.C.: GPO.

———. 1983. "Health Care's Soaring Costs." *New York Times*, 26 August, p. D2.

———. 1986. "The Changing Health Marketplace: Making Life Better or Worse for Americans?" Paper presented at the National Debate on Health Care sponsored by the Texas Department of Human Services, Dallas, 21 April.

Davis, K., G. F. Anderson, S. C. Renn, D. Rowland, C. J. Schramm, and E. P. Steinberg. 1985. "Is Cost Containment Working?" *Health Affairs* 4 (Fall): 81–94.

Davis, K., G. F. Anderson, and E. P. Steinberg. 1984. "Diagnosis Related Group Prospective Payment: Implications for Health Care and Medical Technology." *Health Policy* 4, no. 2:139–47.

Davis, K., and D. Rowland. 1983. "Uninsured and Underserved: Inequities in Health Care in the U.S." *Milbank Memorial Fund Quarterly* 61, no. 2:149–76.

———. 1986. *Medicare Policy: New Directions for Health and Long-Term Care*. Baltimore: Johns Hopkins University Press.

Davis, K., and C. Schoen. 1978. *Health and the War on Poverty: A Ten-Year Appraisal*. Washington, D.C.: Brookings Institution.

Deacon, R., J. Lubitz, M. Gornick, and M. Newton. 1979. "Analysis of Variations in Hospital Use by Medicare Patients in PSROs, 1974–1977." *Health Care Financing Review* 1, no. 1:79–107.

Decker, D. K. 1981. "Health Maintenance Organizations: Background and Perspective." In *Group and IPA HMOs*, edited by D. L. Mackie and D. K. Decker, pp. 4–5. Rockville, Md.: Aspen Systems.

DeLissovoy, G., T. Rice, D. Ermann, and J. Gabel. 1986. "Preferred Provider Organizations: Today's Models and Tomorrow's Prospects." *Inquiry* 23, no. 1:7–15.

DesHarnais, S. I. 1985. "Enrollment in and Disenrollment from Health Maintenance Organizations by Medicaid Recipients." *Health Care Financing Review* 6, no. 3:39–50.

DesHarnais, S. I., E. Kobrinski, J. Chesney, M. Long, R. Ament, and S. Fleming. 1987. "The Early Effects of the Prospective Payment System on Inpatient Utilization and the Quality of Care." *Inquiry* 24, no. 1:7–16.

Dobson, A., J. G. Grier, R. H. Carolson, F. Davis, L. Kucken, B. Steinhardt, G. Ferry, and G. Allen. 1978. "PSROs: Their Current Status and Their Impact to Date." *Inquiry* 15, no. 2:113–28.

Dolan, D. L., ed. 1985. "Blue Cross and Blue Shield's Personal Care Plan—Physician Forum." *North Carolina Medical Journal* 46, no. 9:451–54.

Donabedian, A. 1980. *Explorations in Quality Assessment and Monitoring*. Volume 1, *The Definition of Quality and Approaches to Its Assessment*. Ann Arbor, Mich.: Health Administration Press.

Dowling, W. 1974. "Prospective Payments for Hospital Reimbursement." *Inquiry* 11, no. 3:168–80.

Dunham, A., J. A. Morone, and W. White. 1982. "Restoring Medical Markets: Implications for the Poor." *Journal of Health Politics, Policy and Law* 7, no. 2:488–501.

Eddy, D. M. 1984. "Variations in Physician Practice: The Role of Uncertainty." *Health Affairs* 3 (Summer): 74–89.

Eggers, P. 1985. "Beneficiary Impact of the Medicare Prospective Payment System." Presentation to the Villers Foundation Roundtable, Washington, D.C., 13 December.

Eisenberg, B. S. 1984. "Diagnosis-related Groups, Severity of Illness and Equitable Reimbursement under Medicare." *Journal of the American Medical Association* 251, no. 5:645–46.

Ellwood, D. 1986. "Medicare Risk Contracting: Promise and Problems." *Health Affairs* 5 (Spring): 183–89.

Ermann, D., and J. Gabel. 1984. "Multi-Hospital Systems: Issues and Empirical Findings." *Health Affairs* 3 (Spring): 50–64.

Esposito, A., M. Hupfer, C. Mason, and D. Rogler. 1982. "Abstracts of State Legislated Hospital Cost Containment Programs." *Health Care Financing Review* 4, no. 2:129–58.

Farley, D. 1985. "Case Mix, Severity of Illness and Utilization of Inpatient Services by Poor and Uninsured Patients." Paper presented at the annual meeting of the American Public Health Association, Washington, D.C., November.

Feder, J. 1977. *Medicare: The Politics of Federal Health Insurance.* Lexington, Mass.: D. C. Heath & Company.

Feder, J., J. Hadley, and R. Mullner. 1984a. "Falling through the Cracks: Poverty, Insurance Coverage, and Hospital Care for the Poor, 1980 and 1982." *Milbank Memorial Fund Quarterly* 62, no. 4:544–66.

———. 1984b. "Poor People and Poor Hospitals: Implications for Public Policy." *Journal of Health Politics, Policy and Law* 9, no. 2:237–50.

Feder, J., and J. Holahan. 1985. "Medicaid Program Evaluation: A Synthesis of Interim Findings." Draft report prepared for the Health Care Financing Administration, U.S. Department of Health and Human Services, March. Machine copy.

Federal Trade Commission. 1983. Advisory Opinion to Health Care Management Associates. File No. 8330005. 8 June.

Feldstein, P. J. 1988. *Health Care Economics.* 3d ed. New York: Wiley.

Fetter, R. B., R. E. Mills, D. C. Riedel, and J. D. Thompson. 1977. "The Application of Diagnosis Specific Cost Profiles to Cost and Reimbursement Control in Hospitals." *Journal of Medical Systems* 1, no. 2:137–49.

Firshein J. 1986. "Medicaid HMO Plans Tackle Quality Questions." 1986. *Hospitals* 60 (20 March): 76, 78.

Fox, P., W. Goldbeck, and J. Spies. 1984. *Health Care Cost Management: Private Sector Initiatives.* Ann Arbor, Mich.: Health Administration Press.

Francis, A. M., L. Polissar, and A. B. Lorenz. 1984. "Case of Patients with Colorectal Cancer: A Comparison of a Health Maintenance Organization and Fee-for-Service Practices." *Medical Care* 22, no. 5:418–29.

Freeland, M., G. F. Anderson, and C. Schendler. 1979. "National Hospital Input Price Index." *Health Care Financing Review* 1, no. 1:37–61.

Friedland, J. 1981. "Individual Practice Associations." In *Group and IPA HMOs,* p. 155. *See* Decker 1981.

Fuchs, V. 1974. *Who Shall Live? Health Economics and Social Choices.* New York: Basic Books.

Gabel, J., and D. Ermann. 1985. "Preferred Provider Organizations: Performance, Problems, and Promise." *Health Affairs* 4 (Spring): 24–40.

Gabel, J., C. Jajich-Toch, G. deLissovoy, T. Rice, and H. Cohen. 1988. "The Changing World of Group Health Insurance." *Health Affairs* 7 (Summer): 48–65.

Galblum, T., and S. Trieger. 1982. "Demonstrations of Alternative Delivery Systems under Medicare and Medicaid." *Health Care Financing Review* 3, no. 3:1–11.

Gardner, S. F., S. Kyzr, and F. Sabatino. 1985. "Big Business Embraces Alternate Delivery." *Hospitals* 59 (16 March): 81–84.

Gaus, C., B. Cooper, and C. Hirschman. 1981. *Contracts in HMO and Fee-for-Service Performance.* New York: Wiley.

Ginsburg, P. 1978. "Inflation and the Economic Stabilization Program." In *Health: A Victim or Cause of Inflation?* pp. 31–51. *See* Altman and Eichenholz 1976.

Ginsburg, P., and F. Sloan. 1984. "Hospital Cost Shifting." *New England Journal of Medicine* 310, no. 14:893–98.

Goff, D. 1980. "The Plight of the Urban Public Hospital." *Journal of Health Politics, Policy and Law* 4, no. 4:657–74.

Gonnella, J. S., and M. J. Goran. 1975. "Quality of Patient Care—A Measurement of Change: The Staging Concept." *Medical Care* 13, no. 6:467–73.

Gornick, M., M. Newton, and C. Hackerman. 1980. "Factors Affecting Differences in Medicare Reimbursements for Physicians' Services." *Health Care Financing Review* 1, no. 4:15–37.

Graves, E., and R. Pokras. 1982. "Expected Principal Source of Payment for Hospital Discharges: United States, 1979." *NCHS Advance Data* 75 (16 February). PHS 82–1250.

Gray, B. H., ed. 1983. *The New Health Care for Profit: Doctors and Hospitals in a Competitive Environment.* Washington, D.C.: National Academy Press.

Group Health Association of America (GHAA). 1988a. *HMO Industry Profile: Benefits, Premiums, and Market Structure.* Washington, D.C.

———. 1988b. *HMO Industry Profile: Financial Performance.* Washington, D.C.

———. 1988c. *HMO Industry Profile: Utilization Patterns.* Washington, D.C.

Gruber, L. R., M. Shadle, and C. L. Polich. 1988. "From Movement to Industry: The Growth of HMOs." *Health Affairs* 7 (Summer): 197–208.

Hadley, J. 1982. *More Medical Care: Better Health?* Washington, D.C.: Urban Institute Press.

———. 1983. "Medicaid Reimbursement of Teaching Hospitals." *Journal of Health Politics, Policy and Law* 7, no. 4:911–26.

Hadley, J., and J. Feder. 1985. "Hospital Cost Shifting and Care for the Uninsured." *Health Affairs* 4 (Fall): 67–80.

Hanft, R. S. 1982. "The Impact of Changes in Federal Policy on Academic Health Centers." *Health Affairs* 1 (Fall): 67–82.

Health Research Institute. 1981. *Health Care Cost Containment: A Second Biennial Survey: Participant Report.* Walnut Creek, Calif.

Hellinger, F. J. 1976. "The Effect of Certificate of Need Legislation on Hospital Investment." *Inquiry* 13, no. 2:187–93.

———. 1987. "Selection Bias in Health Maintenance Organizations: Analysis of Recent Evidence." *Health Care Financing Review* 9, no. 2:55–63.

Herzlinger, R. 1985. "How Companies Tackle Health Care Costs: Part II." *Harvard Business Review* 63, no. 5:108–20.

Herzlinger, R., and D. Calkins. 1986. "How Companies Tackle Health Care Costs: Part III." *Harvard Business Review* 64, no. 1:70–80.

Herzlinger, R., and J. Swartz. 1985. "How Companies Tackle Health Care Costs: Part I." *Harvard Business Review* 63, no. 4:69–81.

Hewitt Associates. 1985. *Salaried Employee Benefits Provided by Major U.S. Employers: A Comparison Study, 1979 through 1984.* Philadelphia.

Hill, I. T. 1984. "Medicaid Eligibility: A Descriptive Report of OBRA, TEFRA, and DEFRA Provisions and State Responses." Working paper prepared for the Health Care Financing Administration, U.S. Department of Health and Human Services. Machine copy.

Himmelstein, D. U., S. Woolhandler, M. Harnly, M. B. Bader, R. Silber, H. D. Backer, and A. Jones. 1984. "Patient Transfers: Medical Practice as Social Triage." *American Journal of Public Health* 74, no. 5:494–96.

"HMOs Protecting Senior Citizens." 1986. *Washington Post,* 7 June, p. A22, col. 1.

Holahan, J. 1987. "The Impact of Alternative Medicaid Hospital Payment Systems on Hospitals' Medicaid Revenues, Admissions, and Lengths of Stay." Working Paper. Washington, D.C.: Urban Institute.

Holmes, D. 1986. Personal communication to E. P. Steinberg, January.

Horn, S. D. 1981. "Validity, Reliability and Implications of an Index of Inpatient Severity of Illness." *Medical Care* 19, no. 3:354–67.

Horn, S. D., R. A. Horn, P. D. Sharkey, R. S. Beall, J. S. Hoff, and B. J. Rosenstein. 1986a. "Misclassification Problems in Diagnosis-related Groups." *New England Journal of Medicine* 314, no. 8:484–87.

———. 1986b. "Severity of Illness within DRGs Homogeneity Study." *Medical Care* 24, no. 3:225–35.

Horn, S. D., R. A. Horn, P. D. Sharkey, and A. F. Chambers. 1985. "Severity of Illness within DRGs: Impact on Prospective Payment." *American Journal of Public Health* 75, no. 10:1195–99.

Horn, S. D., D. N. Schumacher, D. A. Bertram, and P. D. Sharkey. 1981. *Measuring Severity of Illness: Homogeneous Case Mix Groups.* Baltimore: Center for Hospital Finance and Management, Johns Hopkins School of Hygiene and Public Health.

Hornbrook, M. C. 1982. "Hospital Case Mix: Its Definition, Measurement and Use: Part II, Review of Alternative Measures." *Medical Care Review* 39, no. 2:73–123.

———. 1984. "Examination of the AAPCC Methodology in an HMO Prospective Payment Demonstration Project." *Group Health Journal* 5, no. 1:13–21.

Hospital Association of New York State. 1978. *Cost of Regulation: Report of the Task Force on Regulation.* New York.

Howell, J. 1984. "Evaluating the Impact of Certificate-of-Need Regulation Using Measures of Ultimate Outcome: Some Cautions from Experience in Massachusetts." *Health Services Research* 19, no. 5:587–612.

Iglehart, J. K. 1982a. "Health Care and American Business." *New England Journal of Medicine* 306, no. 2:120–24.

———. 1982b. "The New Era of Prospective Payment for Hospitals." *New England Journal of Medicine* 307, no. 20:1288–92.

———.1982c. "New Jersey's Experiment with DRG-based Hospital Reimbursement." *New England Journal of Medicine* 307, no. 26:1655–60.

———. 1983a. "Medicaid Turns to Prepaid Managed Care." *New England Journal of Medicine* 308, no. 16:976–80.

———. 1983b. "Medicare Begins Prospective Payment of Hospitals." *New England Journal of Medicine* 308, no. 23:1428–32.

———. 1984a. "Big Business and Health Care in the Heartland: An Interview with Robert Burnett." *Health Affairs* 3 (Spring): 40–49.

———. 1984b. "For-Profit and Not-for-Profit HMOs on the Move." *New England Journal of Medicine* 310, no. 18:1203–8.

———. 1985a. "Medical Care of the Poor—A Growing Problem." *New England Journal of Medicine* 313, no. 1:59–63.

———. 1985b. "Medicare Turns to HMOs." *New England Journal of Medicine* 312, no. 2:132–36.

———. 1986. "Early Experience with Prospective Payment of Hospitals." *New England Journal of Medicine* 314, no. 22:1460–64.

———. 1987. "Second Thoughts about HMOs for Medicare Patients." *New England Journal of Medicine* 316, no. 23:1487–92.

Institute of Medicine (IOM). 1986. *For-Profit Enterprise in Health Care.* Washington, D.C.: National Academy Press.

Interstudy. 1985a. *HMO Summary, June 1985.* Excelsior, Minn.

———. 1985b. *National HMO Census, 1984.* Excelsior, Minn.

———. 1988. *The Interstudy Edge.* Excelsior, Minn.

Jackson-Beeck, M., and J. H. Kleinman. 1983. "Evidence for Self Selection among Health Maintenance Organization Enrollees." *Journal of the American Medical Association* 250, no. 20:2826–29.

Jencks, S. F., and A. Dobson. 1985. "Strategies for Reforming Medicare's Physician Payments: Physician Diagnosis-related Groups and Other Approaches." *New England Journal of Medicine* 312, no. 23:1492–99.

Johns, L., M. D. Anderson, and R. Derzon. 1985. "Selective Contracting in California: Experience in the Second Year." *Inquiry* 22, no. 4:335–47.

Kidder, D., and D. Sullivan. 1982. "Hospital Payroll Costs, Productivity, and Employment under Prospective Reimbursement." *Health Care Financing Review* 4, no. 2:89–100.

Krystenak, L. 1983. "Prospective Payment for Capital: The Financial Nature of Capital Allowances." *Healthcare Financial Management* 37, no. 10:60–76.

Kusserow, R. P. 1986. "Quality of Care for Medicare Beneficiaries." Testimony before the U.S. Senate Committee on Finance, 3 June. Washington, D.C.: GPO.

Lave, J. R. 1984. "Hospital Reimbursement under Medicare." *Milbank Memorial Fund Quarterly, Health and Society* 62, no. 2:251–78.

Lave, J. R., L. B. Lave, and L. P. Silverman. 1972. "Hospital Cost Estimation Controlling for Case Mix." *Applied Economics* 4, no. 3:165–80.

Law, S. 1974. *Blue Cross: What Went Wrong?* New Haven: Yale University Press.

Lefkowitz, B. 1983. *Health Planning Lessons for the Future.* Rockville, Md.: Aspen Systems.

Lerner, M., and D. Salkever. 1983. "The Shift from Inpatient to Outpatient Care for Four Selected Surgical Procedures under the Philadelphia Blue Cross: Evaluation of a Program." In *Proceedings of the Public Health Conference on Records and Statistics.* Washington, D.C., 23 August.

Levit, K. R., H. Lazenby, D. R. Waldo, and L. M. Davidoff. 1985. "National Health Expenditures, 1984." *Health Care Financing Review* 7, no. 1:1–34.

Lewin and Associates. 1986. "Research Agenda: The Impact of PPS and Capitation on Quality and Access to Care." Background paper prepared for the U.S. Public Health Service, Office of Health Planning and Evaluation, 6 May.

Lewin, L., R. Derzon, and R. Marguilies. 1981. "Investor-Owneds and Nonprofits Differ in Economic Performance." *Hospitals* 55 (1 July): 52–58.

Lewis, K. 1984. "Comparison of Use by Enrolled and Recently Disenrolled Populations in a Health Maintenance Organization." *Health Services Research* 19, no. 1:1–22.

Lipscomb, J., I. Raskin, and J. Eichenholz. 1978. "The Use of Marginal Cost Estimates in Hospital Cost Containment Policy." In *Hospital Cost Containment,* edited by M. Zubkoff. New York: Prodist.

Lohr, K. N., R. H. Brook, G. A. Goldberg, M. R. Chassin, and T. K. Glennan. 1985. "Impact of Medicare Prospective Payment on the Quality of Medical Care: A Research Agenda." Paper prepared for the Health Care Financing Administration, U.S. Department of Health and Human Services. Rand Corporation, March.

Louis Harris and Associates. 1984. *Summary Report—A Report Card on HMOs, 1980–1984.* Prepared for the Henry J. Kaiser Family Foundation. New York: Gannett Publishing Company.

———. 1985. *The Equitable Healthcare Survey III: Corporate Initiatives and Employee Attitudes on Cost Containment.* February-March.

Luft, H. 1978. "How Do Health Maintenance Organizations Achieve Their Savings? Rhetoric and Evidence." *New England Journal of Medicine* 298, no. 24:1336–43.

———. 1980. "Trends in Medical Care Costs: Do HMOs Lower the Rate of Growth?" *Medical Care* 18, no. 1:1–16.

———. 1981. *Health Maintenance Organizations: Dimensions of Performance.* New York: Wiley.

———. 1988. "HMOs and the Quality of Care." *Inquiry* 25, no. 1:147–56.

Luft, H., and Miller, R. H. 1988. "Patient Selection in a Competitive Health System." *Health Affairs* 7 (Summer): 97–119.

Lurie, N., N. Ward, M. Shapiro, and R. H. Brook. 1984. "Termination from Medi-Cal: Does It Affect Health?" *New England Journal of Medicine* 311, no. 7:480–84.

McClure, W. 1984. "On Research Status and Risk-adjusted Capitation Rates." *Inquiry* 21, no. 3:205–13.

Mackie, D. L. 1981. "An Overview of HMOs from the Federal Perspective." In *Group and IPA HMOs*, pp. 37–51. *See* Decker 1981.

McMillan, A., J. Lubitz, and D. Russell. 1987. "Medicare Enrollment in Health Maintenance Organizations." *Health Care Financing Review* 8, no. 3:87–93.

McNamara-Bennett, J. 1985. "National HMO Chains on the Rise." *Internist* 26, no. 9:16.

Manning, W. G., A. Liebowitz, G. A. Goldberg, W. H. Rogers, and J. P. Newhouse. 1984. "A Controlled Trial of the Effect of a Prepaid Group Practice on the Use of Services." *New England Journal of Medicine* 310, no. 23:1505–10.

Marmor, T. R. 1973. *The Politics of Medicare.* Chicago: Aldine.

Martin, J., D. Dolkart, and D. Freko. 1984. "Reasons for the Downturn in Under 65 Admissions." Office of Public Policy Analysis Policy Brief No. 52. Chicago: American Hospital Association, 21 September.

Martin, S., M. Schwartz, B. Whalen, D. D'Arpa, G. M. Ljung, J. H. Thorne, and A. E. McKusick. 1982. "Impact of a Mandatory SecondOpinion Program on Medicaid Surgery Rates." *Medical Care* 20, no. 1:21–45.

Mechanic, D., N. Weiss, and P. D. Cleary. 1983. "The Growth of HMOs: Issues of Enrollment and Disenrollment." *Medical Care* 21, no. 93:338–47.

"Medicaid HMO Plans Tackle Quality Questions." 1986. *Hospitals* 60 (20 March): 76–78.

Medical World News, 5 May 1986, p. 16.

Merriam, I. A. 1964. Testimony before the U.S. Senate Special Committee on Aging, Subcommittee on Health of the Elderly, Hearing on Blue Cross and Other Private Health Insurance for the Elderly. S. Doc. 88:2, pp. 3–13. Washington, D.C.

Merrill, J. C. 1984. "Diagnosis Related Groups: Their Role in the Reimbursement System." *Bulletin of the New York Academy of Medicine* 60, no. 5:514–24.

Merrill, J. C., and R. J. Wassermann. 1985. "Growth in National Expenditures: Additional Analyses." *Health Affairs* 4 (Winter): 91–98.

Merritt, R. E. 1986. *State Health Notes.* Washington, D.C.: Intergovernmental Health Policy Project.

Meyer, J. A., and W. R. Johnson. 1983. "Cost Shifting in Health Care: An Economic Analysis." *Health Affairs* 2 (Summer): 20–35.

Mick, S. S., S. Sussman, L. Anderson-Selling, C. DelNero, R. Glazer, E. Hirsch, and D. Rowe. 1983. "Physician Turnover in Eight New England Prepaid Group Practices: An Analysis." *Medical Care* 21, no. 3:323–37.

Mitchell, S. A. 1982. "Issues, Evidence, and the Policymaker's Dilemma." *Health Affairs* 1 (Summer): 84–98.

Mullner, R., and J. Hadley. 1984. "Interstate Variations in the Growth of Chain-owned Proprietary Hospitals, 1973–1982." *Inquiry* 21, no. 2:144–51.

Mulstein, S. 1984. "The Uninsured and Financing of Uncompensated Care: Scope, Costs, and Policy Options." *Inquiry* 21, no. 3:214–29.

Muse, D. N. 1987. "Medicaid Trends: Past, Present, and Future." Presentation to National Health Policy Forum, Washington, D.C., January.

Myerowitz, P. D. 1985. Letter to the Editor. *New England Journal of Medicine* 313, no. 9:583.

National Industrial Council for HMO Development. 1984. *The Health Maintenance Organization Industry Ten Year Report, 1973–1983.* Washington, D.C.

Neuschler, E. 1985a. "Overview of Medicaid Managed Health Care Initiatives." Testimony before the Maryland House of Delegates Appropriations Subcommittee on Health and the Environment, 14 August.

———. 1985b. *Prepaid Managed Care under Medicaid: Overview of Current Initiatives.* Washington, D.C.: National Governors' Association.

Newhouse, J. P., W. G. Manning, C. Morris, L. Orr, N. Dvan, E. B. Keeler, A. Leibowitz, K. Marquis, M. S. Marquis, C. E. Phelps, R. H. Brook. 1981. "Some Interim Results from a Controlled Trial of Cost Sharing in Health Insurance." *New England Journal of Medicine* 305, no. 25:1501–7.

Newhouse, J. P., W. B. Schwartz, A. P. Williams, and C. Witsberger. 1985. "Are Fee-for-Service Costs Increasing Faster then HMO Costs?" *Medical Care* 23, no. 8:960–66.

Okun, A. M. 1975. *Equality and Efficiency: The Big Tradeoff.* Washington, D.C.: Brookings Institution.

Olinger, L. 1986. "Medicaid Program Evaluation: Interim Findings—Inpatient Hospital Reimbursement." Cambridge, Mass.: Abt Associates.

Omenn, G. S., and D. A. Conrad. 1984. "Implications of DRGs for Clinicians." *New England Journal of Medicine* 311, no. 20:1314–17.

"Outlook Good for For-Profit HMOs: Analyst." 1985. *Hospitals* 59 (16 March): 36.

Parker, T. 1988. Health Care Financing Administration. Division of Medicaid Statistics. Personal communication, September.

Pattison, R., and H. Katz. 1983. "Investor-owned and Not-for-Profit Hospitals: A Comparison Based on California Data." *New England Journal of Medicine* 309, no. 6:347–53.

Petersdorf, R. 1985. "A Proposal for Financing Graduate Medical Education." *New England Journal of Medicine* 312, no. 20:1322–24.

Pettingill, J., and J. Vertrees. 1982. "Reliability and Validity in Hospital Case Mix Measurement." *Health Care Financing Review* 4, no. 2:101–28.

"PPOs Face Antitrust Problems." 1984. *Washington Report on Medicine and Health.* Washington, D.C.: McGraw Hill, 5 November.

"PROs: The Future Agenda." 1985. A Report of the American Medical Peer Review Association's Task Force on PRO Implementation. September.

Relman, A. S. 1985. "Economic Considerations in Emergency Care: What Are Hospitals For?" *New England Journal of Medicine* 312, no. 6:372–73.

———. 1986. "Texas Eliminates Dumping." *New England Journal of Medicine* 314, no. 9:578–79.

Renn, S. C., C. J. Schramm, J. M. Watt, and R. Degan. 1985. "The Effects of Ownership System Affiliation on the Economic Performance of Hospitals." *Inquiry* 22, no. 3:219–36.

Rice, T., G. deLissovoy, J. Gabel, and D. Ermann. 1985. "The State of PPOs: Results from a National Survey." *Health Affairs* 4 (Winter):25–40.

Robert Wood Johnson Foundation. 1982. *Affordable Health Care Programs*. Princeton, March.

Rosenberg, R., and D. L. Mackie. 1981. "Physicians in Prepaid Group Practices." In *Group and IPA HMOs*, pp. 109–25. See Decker 1981.

Rossiter, L., and K. Langwell. 1988. "Medicare's Two Systems for Paying Providers." *Health Affairs* 7 (Summer): 120–32.

Rowland, D. 1987. "Hospital Care for the Poor and Uninsured." Ph.D. diss., Johns Hopkins University School of Hygiene and Public Health.

Rowland, D., and B. Lyons. 1987. "Mandatory HMO Care for Milwaukee's Poor." *Health Affairs* 6 (Spring): 87–100.

Rowland, D., B. Lyons, and J. Edwards. 1988. "Medicaid: Health Care for the Poor in the Reagan Era." *Annual Review of Public Health* 9 (Spring): 427–50.

Ruchlin, H., M. L. Finkel, and E. McCarthy. 1982. "The Efficacy of Second-Opinion Consultation Programs." *Medical Care* 20, no. 1:3.

Rundal, T. G., and W. K. Limbert. 1984. "The Private Management of Public Hospitals." *Health Services Research* 15, no. 4:519–44.

Salkever, D., and T. Bice. 1979. "The Impact of Certificate of Need Controls on Hospital Investment." *Milbank Memorial Fund Quarterly* 54, no. 2:185–214.

Sapolsky, H., D. Altman, R. Greene, and J. Moore. 1981. "Corporate Attitudes toward Health Care Costs." *Milbank Memorial Fund Quarterly, Health and Society* 59, no. 4:561–85.

Schaller, D., A. Bostrom, and J. Rafferty. 1986. "Quality of Care Review: Recent Experience in Arizona." *Health Care Financing Review*, annual suppl., pp. 65–74.

Schiff, R., D. Ansell, J. Schlosser, A. Idris, A. Morrison, and S. Whitman. 1986. "Transfers to a Public Hospital: A Prospective Study of 467 Patients." *New England Journal of Medicine* 314, no. 9:552–57.

Schramm, C. J., and J. Gabel. 1988. "Prospective Payment: Some Retrospective Observations." *New England Journal of Medicine* 318, no. 25:1681–83.

Schramm, C. J., S. C. Renn, and B. Biles. 1986. "Controlling Hospital Cost Inflation: New Perspectives on State Rate Setting." *Health Affairs* 5 (Fall): 22–33.

Schramm, C. J., S. C. Renn, J. A. Patrick, G. Lessing, and R. Cohen. 1987. *A Study of the Cost-Effectiveness of Medicare Waivers and the Efficacy of State All Payer Hospital Systems*. Report submitted to the Coalition on State All Payer Hospital Payment Systems, Health Insurance Association of America. Washington, D.C., 28 August.

Schweiker, R. S. 1982. *Report to Congress on Hospital Prospective Payment for Medicare*. Washington, D.C.

———. 1983. "Hospital Prospective Payment for Medicare." Testimony before the U.S. Senate Committee on Finance, Subcommittee on Health. Washington, D.C.: GPO.

Sherlock, D. B. 1986. *For-Profit Prepaid Health Plans: Trends and Financing Implications*. New York: Salomon Brothers.

Simborg, D. W. 1981. "DRG Creep: A New Hospital Acquired Disease." *New England Journal of Medicine* 34, no. 26:1602–4.

Siu, A., A. Leibowitz, R. H. Brook, N. Goldman, N. Lurie, and J. P. Newhouse. 1988. "Use of the Hospital in a Randomized Trial of Prepaid Care." *Journal of the American Medical Association* 259, no. 9:1343–46.

Siu, A., S. A. Sonnenberg, W. G. Manning, G. A. Goldberg, E. S. Blumfield, J. P. Newhouse, and R. H. Brook. 1986. "Inappropriate Use of Hospitals in a Randomized Trial of Health Insurance Plans." *New England Journal of Medicine* 315, no. 20:1259–66.

Sloan, F. 1981. "Regulation and the Rising Cost of Hospital Care." *Review of Economics and Statistics* 63, no. 4:479–87.

———. 1983. "Rate Regulation as a Strategy for Hospital Cost Control: Evidence from the Last Decade." *Milbank Memorial Fund Quarterly* 61, no. 2:195–221.

Sloan, F., and E. R. Becker. 1984. "Cross Subsidies and Payment for Hospital Care." *Journal of Health Politics, Policy and Law* 8, no. 4:660–85.

Sloan, F., R. Feldman, and B. Steinwald. 1983. "Effects of Teaching on Hospital Costs." *Journal of Health Economics* 2, no. 1:1–28..

Sloan, F., and B. Steinwald. 1980a. "Effects of Regulation on Hospital Costs and Input Use." *Journal of Law and Economics* 23, no. 1:81–109.

———. 1980b. *Insurance, Regulation, and Hospital Costs.* Lexington, Mass.: D. C. Heath & Company.

Sloan, F., J. Valvona, and R. Mullner. 1986. "Identifying the Issues: A Statistical Profile." In *Uncompensated Hospital Care: Rights and Responsibilities,* edited by F. Sloan, J. F. Blumstein, and J. M. Perrin. Baltimore: Johns Hopkins University Press.

Sloan, F., and R. A. Vraciu. 1983. "Investor-owned and Not-for-Profit Hospitals: Addressing Some Issues." *Health Affairs* 2 (Spring): 25–37.

Social Security Administration. 1985. *Annual Statistical Supplement, 1984–1985.* Washington, D.C.

Sorenson, A. A., and R. P. Wersinger. 1981. "Factors Influencing Disenrollment from an HMO." *Medical Care* 19, no. 7:766–73.

Starr, P. 1982. *The Social Transformation of American Medicine.* New York: Basic Books.

Stein, J. 1985. "Industry's New Bottom Line on Health Care Costs: Is Less Better?" *Hastings Center Report* 5, no. 5:14–18.

Steinberg, E. P., and D. M. Hynes. 1986. "A Case Study of HMO Development in Baltimore—Implications for National Trends." Working Paper, Johns Hopkins Center for Hospital Finance and Management.

Steinwald, B., and F. Sloan. 1981. "Regulatory Approaches to Hospital Cost Containment: A Synthesis of the Empirical Evidence." In *A New Approach to the Economics of Health Care,* edited by M. Olson, pp. 275–308. Washington, D.C.: American Enterprise Institute.

Stern, R. S., and A. M. Epstein. 1985. "Institutional Responses to Prospective Payment Based on Diagnosis-related Groups." *New England Journal of Medicine* 312, no. 10:621–27.

Strumpf, G. B. 1981. "Historical Evolution and the Political Process." In *Group and IPA HMOs,* pp. 17–19. *See* Decker 1981.

Sulvetta, M., and K. Swartz. 1986. *The Uninsured and Uncompensated Care: A Chartbook.* Washington, D.C.: National Health Policy Forum, June.

Swartz, W., J. P. Newhouse, and A. P. Williams. 1985. "Is the Teaching Hospital an Endangered Species?" *New England Journal of Medicine* 313, no. 3:157–62.

Tell, E., M. Falik, and P. Fox. 1984. "Private-Sector Health Care Initiatives: A Comparative Perspective from Four Communities." *Milbank Memorial Fund Quarterly* 62, no. 3:357–79.

Thomas, J. W., S. E. Berki, R. Lichtenstein, and L. Wyszewianski. 1984. "A Health Status Measure for Adjusting the HMO Capitation Rates of Medicare Beneficiaries." Final report for Grant No. 18-P–98179/501. Health Care Financing Administration, U.S. Department of Health and Human Services. Washington, D.C.: GPO.

"Title XIII—Health Maintenance Organizations." 1982. In *Compilation of Selected Acts within the Jurisdiction of the House Committee on Energy and Commerce,* vol. 1, *Health Law.* Washington, D.C.: GPO.

Traska, M. R. 1985a. "Baby Boomers Help HMOs Grow to 42 States." *Hospitals* 59 (16 May): 84, 88–89.

———. 1985b. "Outlook Good for For-Profit HMOs: Analyst." *Hospitals* 59 (16 March): 36.

Trieger, S., T. Galblum, and G. Riley. 1981. "HMOs: Issues and Alternatives for Medicare and Medicaid." Health Care Financing Administration Publication No. 03107. Baltimore, April. Machine copy.

U.S. Chamber of Commerce. 1985. *Employee Benefits, 1984.* Washington, D.C.

U.S. Congress. 1973. *Health Maintenance Organization Act (Title XIII of the Public Health Service Act).* 93d Cong., 1st sess.

———. 1982. *Tax Equity and Fiscal Responsibility Act of 1982 (TEFRA).* 97th Cong., 2d sess. PL 97–248.

———. 1983. *Social Security Act Amendments of 1983.* 98th Cong., 1st sess. PL 98–21.

U.S. Congress. Congressional Budget Office (CBO). 1979a. *Controlling Rising Hospital Costs.* Washington, D.C.: GPO.

———. 1979b. *The Effect of PSROs on Health Care Costs: Current Findings and Future Evaluations.* Washington, D.C.: GPO.

———. 1981. *The Impact of PSROs on Health Care Costs: An Update of CBO's 1979 Evaluation.* Washington, D.C.: GPO.

———. 1986. *Physician Reimbursement under Medicare: Options for Change.* Washington, D.C.: GPO, April.

U.S. Congress. House. Committee on Energy and Commerce. 1986. *Statement to the Committee on the Budget regarding the Administration's FY 1987 Budget.* Washington, D.C., March.

U.S. Congress. House. Committee on Ways and Means. 1987. *Background Material and Data on Programs within the Jurisdiction of the Committee on Ways and Means.* WMCP 100–4. 100th Cong., 1st sess. Washington, D.C.: GPO.

———. 1988. *Background Material and Data on Programs Within the Jurisdiction of the Committee on Ways and Means.* WMCP 100–29. 100th Cong., 2d sess. Washington, D.C.: GPO.

U.S. Congress. Office of Technology Assessment (OTA). 1986. *Payment for Physician Services: Strategies for Medicare*. Washington, D.C.: GPO.

U.S. Congress. Prospective Payment Assessment Commission (ProPAC). 1985. *1986 Adjustments to the Medicare Prospective Payment System: Report to the Congress*. Washington, D.C.: GPO, November.

———. 1986. *Technical Appendixes to the Report and Recommendations to the Secretary, U.S. Department of Health and Human Services*. Washington, D.C.: GPO, 1 April.

———. 1989. *Report and Recommendations to the Secretary, U.S. Department of Health and Human Services*. Washington, D.C.: GPO, 1 March.

U.S. Congress. Senate. Committee on Finance. 1983. *Social Security Amendments of 1983*. Washington, D.C.: GPO, 11 March.

———. 1986. *Quality and Access to Health Care under Medicare's Prospective Payment System*. 99th Cong., 2d sess. Background paper, May.

U.S. Congress. Senate. Special Committee on Aging. 1985. *Impact of Medicare's Prospective Payment System on the Quality of Care Received by Medicare Beneficiaries*. 99th Cong., 1st sess. Staff report, 23 September.

U.S. Congress. Social Security Advisory Council. 1984. *Medicare Benefits and Financing: Report of the 1982 Advisory Council on Social Security to the Secretary, Department of Health and Human Services*. 98th Cong., 2d sess. February.

U.S. Department of Commerce. Bureau of the Census (Census). 1985. "Economic Characteristics of Households in the United States: Fourth Quarter, 1983." *Current Population Reports*, ser. P-70-83-4. Washington, D.C.

———. 1986. "Estimates of the Population of the United States to March 1, 1986." *Current Population Reports*, ser. P-25-86-1, no. 987. Washington, D.C., June.

———. 1987a. "Economic Characteristics of Households in the United States." *Current Population Reports*, ser. P-60-87-1. Washington, D.C.

———. 1987b. *Statistical Abstract of the United States, 1987*. Washington, D.C.

U.S. Department of Health and Human Services (DHHS). 1980. *Federal Register*.

———. 1985. "Medicare Program: Changes to the Inpatient Hospital Prospective Payment System and Fiscal Year 1986 Rates: Final Rules." *Federal Register* 50:35722.

———. 1988. *Monthly Vital Statistics Report* 37:1.

U.S. Department of Health and Human Services. Health Care Financing Administration (HCFA). 1982. *Medicare and Medicaid Data Book, 1981*. Baltimore: Office of Research and Demonstrations.

———. 1985. *Analysis of State Medicaid Program Characteristics, 1984*. Baltimore: Office of Research and Demonstrations.

———. 1986a. *Medicare and Medicaid Data Book, 1984*. Baltimore: Office of Research and Demonstrations.

———. 1986b. *Report to Congress: Impact of the Medicare Hospital Prospective Payment System, 1984 Report*, HCFA Pub. No. 03231. Washington, D.C.

———. 1987a. *Analysis of State Medicaid Program Characteristics, 1986*. Baltimore: Office of Research and Demonstrations.

———. 1987b. "National Health Expenditures, 1986–2000." *Health Care Financing Review* 8, no. 4:1–36.

———. 1988. Data Evaluation Report, June.

U.S. Department of Health and Human Services. Office of Health Maintenance Organizations (OHMO). 1983. *The 1983 Investors Guide to Health Maintenance Organizations.* Washington, D.C.: Touche Ross & Co., June.

———. 1985a. "Data on For Profit Operational Prepaid Health Care Plans in the U.S., 15 December." Computer printout.

———. 1985b. "Statistical Data for the Type A Federally Qualified HMO Population of the United States of America, 3rd Quarter." Computer printout.

U.S. Department of Health, Education, and Welfare (DHEW). 1971. *Towards a Comprehensive Health Policy for the 1970s: A White Paper.* Washington, D.C.

U.S. Department of Justice. 1984. *Federal Register* 49:26823–37.

U.S. Department of Labor. Bureau of Labor Statistics. 1988. *Economic Report of the President.* Washington, D.C.: GPO.

U.S. General Accounting Office (GAO). 1985a. *Information Requirements for Evaluating the Impacts of Medicare Prospective Payment on Post-Hospital Long-Term Care Services: Preliminary Report.* GAO/PEMD-85-8. Washington, D.C., February.

———. 1985b. *Use of Unaudited Hospital Cost Data Resulted in Overstatement of Medicare's Prospective Payment Rate.* GAO/HRD-85-74. Washington, D.C., 18 July.

———. 1986. *Medicare: Issues Raised by Florida Health Maintenance Organization Demonstrations.* GAO/HRD-86-97. Washington, D.C., July.

Vladeck, B. 1981. "Equity, Access, and the Costs of Health Services." *Medical Care* 19, no. 12, suppl.: 69–79.

———. 1984. "Medicare Hospital Payment by Diagnosis-related Groups." *Annals of Internal Medicine* 100, no. 4:576–91.

Ware, J. E., R. H. Brook, W. H. Rogers, E. B. Keeler, A. R. Davies, C. D. Sherbourne, G. A. Goldberg, P. Camp, and J. P. Newhouse. 1986. "Comparison of Health Outcomes at 9 Health Maintenance Organizations with Those of Fee-for-Service Care." *Lancet* 1, no. 8488:1017–22.

Weiner, S. 1977. "Reasonable Cost Reimbursement for Inpatient Hospital Services under Medicare and Medicaid: The Emergence of Public Control." *American Journal of Law and Medicine* 3, no. 1:1–48.

Wennberg, J. 1984. "Dealing with Medical Practice Variations: A Proposal for Action." *Health Affairs* 3 (Summer): 6–32.

———. 1986. "Which Rate Is Right?" *New England Journal of Medicine* 314, no. 5:310–11.

———. 1987. "The Paradox of Appropriate Care." *Journal of the American Medical Association* 258, no. 18:2568–69.

Wennberg, J., and A. Gittlesohn. 1975. "Health Care Delivery in Maine: I. Patterns of Use of Common Surgical Procedures." *Journal of the Maine Medical Association* 66:123–30.

———. 1982. "Variations in Medical Care among Small Areas." *Scientific American* 246:120–34.

Wennberg, J., K. McPherson, and P. Caper. 1984. "Will Payment Based on Diagnosis-related Groups Control Hospital Costs?" *New England Journal of Medicine* 311, no. 5:295–300.

Whitney, S. 1985. U.S. Department of Health and Human Services, Office of Health Maintenance Organizations. Personal communication, December.

Wilensky, G. 1984. "Solving Uncompensated Hospital Care: Targeting the Indigent and the Uninsured." *Health Affairs* 3 (Winter): 50–62.

Wood, D. 1988. Health Care Financing Administration. Division of Information Analysis. Personal communication to E. P. Steinberg. September.

Worthington, N. L., and P. A. Piro. 1982. "The Effects of Hospital Rate-setting Programs on Volumes of Hospital Services: A Preliminary Analysis." *Health Care Financing Review* 4, no. 2:47–66.

Wrenn, K. 1985. "No Insurance, No Admission." *New England Journal of Medicine* 312, no. 6:373–74.

Yelin, E. H., C. J. Hienke, J. S. Kramer, M. C. Nevitt, M. Shearn, and W. V. Epstein. 1985. "A Comparison of the Treatment of Rheumatoid Arthritis in Health Maintenance Organizations and Fee-for-Service Practices." *New England Journal of Medicine* 312, no. 15:962–67.

Young, W. W. 1979. "Measuring the Cost of Care Using Generalized Patient Management Paths." Progress Report for Grant No. 18-p97063/3d, submitted to the Health Care Financing Administration, November.

Young, W. W., R. B. Swinkola, and D. M. Zorn. 1982. "The Measurement of Hospital Case Mix," *Medical Care* 20, no. 5:501–12.

Index